MEDICAL INNOVATION AT THE CROSSROADS

D1267868

VOLUME III

Technology and Health Care

in

An Era of Limits

Annetine C. Gelijns, Editor

Committee on Technological Innovation in Medicine
INSTITUTE OF MEDICINE

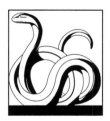

National Academy Press
Washington, D.C. 1992

NATIONAL ACADEMY PRESS • 2101 Constitution Avenue, N.W. • Washington, D.C. 20418

The Institute of Medicine was chartered in 1970 by the National Academy of Sciences to enlist distinguished members of the appropriate professions in the examination of policy matters pertaining to the health of the public. In this the Institute acts under both the Academy's 1863 congressional charter responsibility to be an advisor to the federal government and its own initiative in identifying issues of medical care, research, and education.

The Committee on Technological Innovation in Medicine was established in 1988 by the Institute of Medicine to design a series of workshops that would (a) provide more fundamental knowledge of the process by which biomedical research findings are translated into clinical practice and (b) address opportunities for improving the rationality and efficiency of the process. This volume consists of the proceedings of the third workshop in the series, "The Changing Health Care Economy: Impact on Physicians, Patients, and Innovators," held April 18–19, 1991. This workshop and its proceedings were supported by the Howard Hughes Medical Institute, Pfizer, Inc., and the Health Industry Manufacturers Association. The opinions and conclusions expressed here are those of the authors and do not necessarily represent the views of the National Academy of Sciences or any of its constituent parts.

Library of Congress Cataloging-in-Publication Data

Technology and health care in an era of limits / Annetine C. Gelijns,
    editor ; Committee on Technological Innovation in Medicine,
    Institute of Medicine.
        p. cm . — (Medical innovation at the crossroads ; v. 3)
    Proceedings of a workshop held April 18–19, 1991, supported by the
    Howard Hughes Medical Institute, Pfizer, Inc., and the Health
    Industry Manufacturers Association.
    Includes bibliographical references and index.
    ISBN 0-309-04695-5
    1. Managed care plans (Medical care) —Congresses. 2. Medical
    care—United States—Congresses. I. Gelijns, Annetine.
    II. Institute of Medicine (U.S.). Committee on Technological
    Innovation in Medicine. III. Howard Hughes Medical Institute.
    IV. Pfizer Inc. V. Health Industry Manufacturers Association.
    VI. Series.
    [DNLM: 1. Cross-Cultural Comparison—congresses. 2. Delivery of
    Health Care—United States—congresses. 3. Health Policy—United
    States—congresses. 4. Technology, Medical—congresses. W1 ME342F
    v. 3]
    Ra413.H39   1992
    36.1—dc20
    DNLM/DLC   92-22704
    for Library of Congress   CIP

Available from: National Academy Press, 2101 Constitution Avenue, NW, Washington, D.C. 20418

Copyright 1992 by the National Academy of Sciences
Printed in the United States of America

The serpent has been a symbol of long life, healing, and knowledge among almost all cultures and religions since the beginning of recorded history. The image adopted as a logotype by the Institute of Medicine is based on a relief carving from ancient Greece, now held at the Staatlichemuseen in Berlin.

RA
413
T4
1992

Committee on Technological Innovation in Medicine

GERALD D. LAUBACH, *Chair*, Former President, Pfizer, Inc.
SUSAN BARTLETT FOOTE, Health Advisor, Office of Senator Dave
Durenberger, U.S. Senate
BEN L. HOLMES, Vice President and General Manager, Medical Products
Group, Hewlett-Packard Company
WILLIAM N. HUBBARD, JR., Former President, the Upjohn Company
LUCIAN LEAPE, Lecturer on Health Policy, Harvard School of Public
Health
KENNETH MELMON, Arthur L. Bloomfield Professor of Medicine and
of Pharmacology, Department of Medicine, Stanford University
School of Medicine
H. RICHARD NESSON, President, Brigham and Womens Hospital
UWE E. REINHARDT, James Madison Professor of Political Economy,
Woodrow Wilson School of Public and International Affairs, Princeton
University
NATHAN ROSENBERG, Professor of Economics, Stanford University
MICHAEL SOPER, National Medical Director, CIGNA
JOHN E. WENNBERG, Professor of Epidemiology, Department of
Community and Family Medicine, Dartmouth Medical School

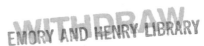

WITHDRAW
EMORY AND HENRY LIBRARY

PROJECT STAFF

Division of Health Care Services

Karl D. Yordy, Director
Kathleen N. Lohr, Deputy Director
Donald Tiller, Administrative Assistant

Program on Technological Innovation in Medicine

Annetine C. Gelijns, Program Director
Holly Dawkins, Research Assistant
Helen Rogers, Senior Project Assistant
Leah Mazade, Staff Editor

Division of Health Sciences Policy

Ruth Ellen Bulger, Director
David Turner, Staff Officer

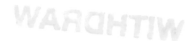

Acknowledgments

The Committee on Technological Innovation in Medicine wishes to acknowledge the many individuals and organizations who contributed to this volume. In particular, we thank John E. Wennberg, who was the main committee member responsible for this project, and without whose guidance and insights this book would not have seen the light of day. The papers in this volume were originally presented at the Institute of Medicine (IOM) workshop, "The Changing Health Care Economy: Impact on Physicians, Patients, and Innovators" (see Appendix A). The committee greatly appreciates the opportunity provided by the Howard Hughes Medical Institute, Pfizer, Inc., and the Health Industry Manufacturers Association to investigate the dynamics of technological innovation in medicine. It also recognizes the significant contributions of the moderators, discussants, and workshop participants to the issues discussed here.

Finally, and in particular, the committee would like to express its gratitude to the IOM staff who facilitated the work of the committee. We especially thank Annetine C. Gelijns, who directs the program on technological innovation in medicine, for her assistance in conceptualizing and editing this volume. The committee also appreciates the support of David Turner and Ruth Ellen Bulger, respectively staff officer and director of the Division of Health Sciences Policy, in organizing and shaping the workshop. Holly Dawkins provided excellent substantive and procedural contributions to the committee's work. We are also grateful for the logistical support and manuscript preparation provided by Helen Rogers. The manuscript's final form owes a great deal to the thorough copyediting of Leah Mazade. Among other IOM members who contributed to this publication are Kathleen N. Lohr, deputy director of the Division of Health Care Services, Karl D. Yordy, director of the Division of Health Care Services, Richard A. Rettig, senior staff officer of the Division of Health Sciences Policy, and executive officer Enriqueta Bond.

GERALD D. LAUBACH
Chair
Committee on Technological
Innovation in Medicine

Contents

List of Abbreviations

ABMT	autologous bone marrow transplantation
ACS	American Cancer Society
ADRDA	Alzheimer's Disease and Related Disorders Association
AIDS	acquired immune deficiency syndrome
AHCPR	Agency for Health Care Policy and Research
AMA	American Medical Association
BPH	benign prostatic hyperplasia
CNS	central nervous system
CON	certificate of need
COP	Committee on Prevention, Group Health Cooperative of Puget Sound
CPT	Current Procedural Terminology
CPT-4	Current Procedural Terminology, 4th edition
CSS	Cancer Surveillance System
CT	computed tomography
DON	determination of need (in Massachusetts)
DRG	diagnosis-related group
ECG	electrocardiogram
FDA	Food and Drug Administration
FTEs	full-time-equivalent employees
GHC	Group Health Cooperative of Puget Sound
GNP	gross national product
GP	general practitioner

HCA	Hospital Corporation of America
HCFA	Health Care Financing Administration
HMO	health maintenance organization
HP	Hewlett-Packard
ICD-9	International Classification of Disease, 9th edition
ICI	Imperial Chemical Industries
ICU	intensive care unit
IND	investigational new drug
IOM	Institute of Medicine
IPA	independent practice association
MRI	magnetic resonance imaging
MS	multiple sclerosis
NHS	National Health Service, United Kingdom
NIH	National Institutes of Health
PMA	premarket approval
PORTs	patient outcome research teams
POS	point of service
PPRC	Physician Payment Review Commission
PPS	Prospective Payment System
PTCA	percutaneous transluminal coronary angioplasty
QALY	quality-adjusted life year
R&D	research and development
RBRVS	resource-based relative value scale
RCT	randomized, controlled clinical trial
t-PA	tissue plasminogen activator
UCLA	University of California, Los Angeles
VHA	Voluntary Hospitals of America

Part I
Setting the Stage

1

Introduction

Gerald D. Laubach, John E. Wennberg, and Annetine C. Gelijns

This volume summarizes the third of a series of Institute of Medicine (IOM) workshops whose intent is to critically examine medical innovation—that is, the process by which medical research findings are translated into actual benefits in clinical practice. The raison d'être for this third workshop (see Appendix A) is deftly captured in the opening sentence of the second chapter: "The U.S. health care sector is the target of a massive social struggle over its reform." Our purpose here is not to become additional participants in that debate but rather to visualize the restructured U.S. health care system that might ultimately emerge from it. In that visualization, we are particularly interested in the likely implications of the new system for practitioners, patients, and the generators of new medical technology.

Such an undertaking inevitably involves a good deal of speculation. On closer examination, however, the degree of speculation may not be nearly as great as one might anticipate. Although currently more than two dozen discrete proposals for restructuring health care in the United States have been put forward, many of them seem transitional in nature. Workshop participants seemed to agree that two alternative scenarios of health care financing and delivery stand out as likely candidates. The first mirrors an extension of current trends: a mature form of today's pluralistic public-private system that relies heavily on managed care to influence ("micromanage") physician and patient decision making directly. The second sce-

3

nario reflects more radical reform: the creation of a system that allows the public sector to set global limits on health care (which might be characterized as "macromanagement").

If these very different scenarios are, indeed, the two most probable ones, assessing their implications becomes a more manageable task. Managed care, mediated through the array of techniques described in this volume, has already become a prominent feature of the American medical landscape (see the papers by Soper and Ferriss, and Welch and Fisher). "Global limit" systems are well established in many nations; this volume discusses Canada—as an example of a social insurance-based system—and the United Kingdom—as an example of a national health system—in detail (see Barer and Evans, and Williams). In the United States, the "classic" health maintenance organization (HMO) can be classified as a subsystem that manages care by setting global limits (see Wagner, in this volume). The perceived impact of the above-mentioned contrasting scenarios on physicians, patients, hospital administrators, and innovators—and on their decisions to adopt, use, or generate new medical interventions—is the principal subject matter of the papers in this volume. Before turning to these papers, it might be useful to discuss briefly the earlier work of the committee, which provides an important foundation for the present discussion.

Because economic concerns are one of the principal factors driving health care reform, it is not surprising that economic constraints on innovation are perceived as a highly probable consequence of any plausible scenario for the evolving system of U.S. health care. The significant influence of economic pressures on both the rate and direction of medical innovation is amply documented in the second volume of this series. Both foreign global limit schemes and evolving managed care practices in the United States tend to discourage the acceptance of new technologies and to control their pricing—thus reducing the economic incentives for innovation as well as the resources for continuing research and development (R&D) efforts. At the same time, health care systems that prize efficiency create an environment that is favorable to particular kinds of innovative activities. For example, it is instructive to note that laparoscopic cholecystectomy, percutaneous transluminal coronary angioplasty (PTCA), and the lithotripter, all of which provide alternatives to costly clinical procedures, originated in Europe. Papers in this volume (see Telling, Holmes, and Moody) report that the growth of managed care practices is stimulating a stronger focus on the development of cost-effective technology as an explicit R&D target. Moreover, pharmaceutical and device firms are investing more in quality-of-life and cost-effectiveness analyses to demonstrate the clinical and economic advantages of these new technologies.

What may be even more important is that cost-conscious health care systems seem to instill a more balanced appreciation of the variations in cost and cost-effectiveness within the vast range of medical technologies (see also the papers by Griner and Hillman). This volume defines the term *medical technology* broadly to encompass medical devices, instrumentation, pharmaceuticals, biologicals, diagnostic and therapeutic procedures, and integrated systems of care delivery. This definition is at variance with the stereotype of medical technology as being inherently and invariably cost inflating. Some medical interventions, such as organ transplants, are indeed quite expensive (albeit potentially cost-effective); yet the cost of one of the most cost-effective technologies, the poliomyelitis vaccine, is trivial. Discrimination among existing alternative technologies to ensure their appropriate use, as well as encouragement of the development of cost-effective new interventions, seems a logical goal of all health care systems.

Beyond these relatively straightforward economic considerations, our earlier workshops have revealed other vulnerabilities of the innovation process that could become acute in cost-sensitive health care systems. One is the tendency to discourage experimentation, both with regard to the use of emerging technologies and the exploration of new uses for accepted technologies. The consequences may be serious, because innovation takes place not only in academic and industrial laboratories but also at the bedside. Small departures from established practice have yielded several important advances, a process that has produced substantial progress in surgery. But the phenomenon applies as well to technologies that are the end result of elaborate, formal R&D processes, such as those employed in the development of pharmaceuticals. A case in point is the evolution of adrenergic beta-blocking drugs, one of the more significant medical innovations of our time. These compounds were introduced for the treatment of two cardiovascular indications, arrhythmias and angina pectoris. Today, they are used in the treatment of more than 20 diverse conditions, largely as a result of clinical discoveries made after beta-blockers were in general use (Gelijns and Thier, 1990).

The interweaving of innovation with clinical practice applies not only to the generation or creation of medical interventions but also to their production and delivery. For example, the ways in which products and human processes are packaged into discrete "units" of care—such as a coronary bypass procedure or an intensive care unit (ICU)—may vary substantially between institutions and even among individuals within one institution. In the case of an emerging technology, this is not surprising, given that its optimum manner of use, the clinical results it produces, and the resource costs associated with it may not have stabilized. Even in the case of established technologies, however, their safety, effectiveness, and appropriateness typically depend on who uses them, how skillfully, and in what clinical situation. In contrast to other economic sectors, the "production" processes of medicine have relatively little standardization. Because the evaluative clinical sciences are underdeveloped, the optimum use of many technologies is an unresolved clinical problem (Wennberg, 1990).

This phenomenon underlies an important deficiency of medical technology assessment as it is often practiced. The important contribution to the process of further development and definitive evaluation that can be made by studying the outcomes of a new intervention in actual practice is not often reflected in the technology policies of otherwise sophisticated health care systems. Not infrequently, decision-making processes seem to be based on the idea that a technology can be evaluated, once and for all, on the basis of research findings collected before its use in everyday practice. But such assessments—conducted in carefully controlled clinical settings—often tell us much less than we need to know about the actual performance of a technology. These decision-making processes reflect an idealized, unrealistic understanding of both medical practice and medical innovation.

In sum, previous work of the committee indicates that the net social benefit of some of the anticipated technology policies of a restructured American health care system may be positive. The predictable emphasis on cost-effective technologies, as exemplified by the trend toward minimally invasive procedures, may offer something for everyone: potential economic savings for payers, better-quality care for patients, professional growth for practitioners, and strong encouragement to particular kinds of innovation. The impact of other likely policies may be ambiguous or negative. For example, the systematic discouragement of experimental technologies may actually produce little or no savings in health care expenditures and could well reduce future benefits—both economic and humane—that might have flowed from successful innovation. Indeed, the overarching risk to society of today's technology policies may well be their inherent conservatism—their tendency to "freeze in place the status quo," as Neumann and Weinstein (1991) observed in an earlier volume in this series. Because much of today's medical technology is both costly and limited in its effectiveness—the "halfway technologies" of Lewis Thomas—delaying the emergence of more definitive interventions may be unsound policy.

It is not obvious that health care policies need to dampen innovation to achieve their intended purpose—that is, encouraging cost-effective care. Instead, it may prove possible to devise policies that constructively merge a comprehensive, cost-conscious U.S. health care system with a more rational program in the evaluative clinical sciences—and at the same time preserve a strong commitment to medical research and development. What, then, are some of these policies? Our deliberations to date suggest a few.

1. Adopt the philosophy and techniques of modern industrial practice to foster a process of continuous quality improvement in health care. Such policies systematically and constructively alter the status quo. Moreover,

U.S. private-sector health care firms might be expected to be strongly attracted to the concept, given the widespread interest in continuous improvement strategies in American industry today. Provocative evidence suggests that these techniques can work in medical settings (Berwick et al., 1990). Britain's National Health Service is also exploring reforms along these lines (Berwick et al., 1992a, b).

2. Capitalize on the massive data bases required for accounting purposes in the U.S. health care system by making them an instrument for continuous evaluation of medical practice. Such a strategy would not discourage the new and experimental by denying reimbursement but instead would require participation in a systematic program of evaluation. It would utilize the same principles to reevaluate older, potentially obsolete technologies.

3. Adopt a universal policy of transparency for technology policies and reimbursement decision rules. In the pluralistic U.S. system, such an open policy would help optimize the social benefits of medical technology.

4. Adopt policies that more systematically engage patients in decision making regarding their treatment. This volume strongly supports the ethical case for including the patient as a full partner in clinical practice (see the papers by Mulley and Silberman). Less well recognized is the economic case—some patients prefer more conservative, less costly options for the management of their medical problems than might be chosen by their physicians alone.

5. Finally, incorporate policies that explicitly encourage technological innovation, including adequate evaluation. Numerous countries have successfully implemented public policies to counterbalance the innovation-suppressing effects of health care regulation; for example, the British National Health Service and the French and Japanese governments retain explicit incentives for innovation in their pharmaceutical pricing formulas (Burstall, 1991; Neimeth, 1991). Thus, policies to compensate for unintended suppression of innovation in health care can be crafted, and indications are that they do, indeed, work.

In conclusion, both the United States and the majority of other industrialized nations are actively debating how to reform their health care systems. These debates are generally couched in terms of consequences of changes in health care for costs, access, and quality. Often overlooked are the likely implications of such changes for medical innovation—and the subsequent effect of innovation on costs, access, and quality. It is our hope that the discussions in this volume encourage consideration of these issues.

REFERENCES

Berwick, D. M., Godfrey, A. B., and Roessner, J. 1990. *Curing Health Care.* San Francisco: Jossey-Bass Publishers.

Berwick, D. M., Enthoven, A., and Bunker, J. P. 1992a. Quality management in the NHS: The doctor's role—I. *British Medical Journal* 304:235-239.

Berwick, D. M., Enthoven, A., and Bunker, J. P. 1992b. Quality management in the NHS: The doctor's role—II. *British Medical Journal* 304:304-308.

Burstall, M. L. 1991. European policies influencing pharmaceutical innovation. In: A. C. Gelijns and E. A. Halm, eds. *Medical Innovation at the Crossroads*. Vol. 2, *The Changing Economics of Medical Technology*. Washington, D.C.: National Academy Press, pp. 123-140.

Gelijns, A. C., and Thier, S. O. 1990. Medical technology development: An introduction to the innovation-evaluation nexus. In: A. C. Gelijns, ed. *Medical Innovation at the Crossroads*. Vol. 1, *Modern Methods of Clinical Investigation*. Washington, D.C.: National Academy Press, pp. 1-15.

Neimeth, R. 1991. Japan's pharmaceutical industry postwar evolution. In: A. C. Gelijns and E. A. Halm, eds. *Medical Innovation at the Crossroads*. Vol. 2, *The Changing Economics of Medical Technology*. Washington, D.C.: National Academy Press, pp. 155-167.

Neumann, P. J., and Weinstein, M. C. 1991. The diffusion of new technology: Costs and benefits to health care. In: A. C. Gelijns and E. A. Halm, eds. *Medical Innovation at the Crossroads*. Vol. 2, *The Changing Economics of Medical Technology*. Washington, D.C.: National Academy Press, pp. 21-34.

Wennberg, J. E. 1990. What is outcomes research? In: A. C. Gelijns, ed. *Medical Innovation at the Crossroads*. Vol. 1, *Modern Methods of Clinical Investigation*. Washington, D.C.: National Academy Press, pp. 33-46.

2

Innovation and the Policies of Limits in A Changing Health Care Economy

John E. Wennberg

The U.S. health care sector is the target of a massive social struggle over its reform. The strategies of the past have failed to establish access and contain costs. Indeed, the trend today is toward less access for the poor and many in the middle class, with more care for those who remain "entitled." Thirty-three million Americans are without health insurance. For those with insurance, the rates of utilization of physician services and expensive diagnostic techniques and the number of invasive procedures being performed continue to spiral. If these trends are not altered, the United States will be spending more than 15 percent of its gross national product (GNP) on health by the year 2000. The message of the 1992 presidential debates is that this situation must change. The systems for financing care must be fixed; to do this costs must be contained. Improvements in access must be accompanied by policies of limits.

The way the politics and policies of limits are fashioned will depend on assumptions about the relationship between the utilization of care and the benefits of care—that is, on the shape of the "benefit-utilization curve." One popular interpretation is that the shape of this curve is such that the nation needs to ration effective care. Patient demand and medical progress now make the health care system so expensive that it can no longer be available on equal terms to everyone; moreover, the nation simply cannot afford to pay for everything that works and that patients want. This predicament arises because of the successes of biomedical research, the resulting efficacy of clinical science, and the efficiency of practicing physicians in translating medical knowledge into beneficial medical interventions. As utilization increases, benefits also increase, but at a declining rate of return as the level of invested resources increase. Somewhere along the curve, society finds itself in a zone in which the benefits can no longer be afforded: the costs of further transfers of GNP toward health care and away from national priorities such as education and housing are simply too great. As a consequence, society must learn to make explicit judgments about the value of specific services as they apply to an individual patient's case. Some experts advocate rationing by age; others recommend using detailed algorithms for specific patient subgroups defined on the basis of "cost-effectiveness."[1] The intent, however, is the same. Policies are needed to set limits on specific services, to develop explicit methods to ration effective care that brings less than socially acceptable marginal returns. The effect of such policies is to deny access to care that works and that patients want on the basis that it is not cost-effective. In the opinion of many, this denial of access inevitably produces a two-tiered system of care, one for the affluent and another for those whose access to care must be underwritten by policies of entitlement.

An alternative interpretation emphasizes that the inadequacies of clinical science and flaws in the role of the physician as the decision-making "agent" of the patient make it impossible to determine the shape of the benefit-utilization curve in medicine. Although investments in basic biomedical science have greatly increased the power of technology to intervene in the natural history of disease, efforts to evaluate the outcomes of these interventions—the effects of medical technology and theories of efficacy in the specific situations of everyday practice—have substantially failed. The risks and benefits of most medical care are poorly understood. Moreover, the agency role of the physician is flawed by professional dominance. This role, which depends on the capacity of physicians to make vicarious judgments about what patients want, has created a market in which the preferences of patients are entangled with those of the physician. In short, in medicine, too little is known about what works and what patients want.

This interpretation emphasizes the major role played by supplier-induced demand, in which the weaknesses in the scientific and ethical status of clinical medicine ensure that available resources are utilized without evidence that more is necessarily better or that patients necessarily want

---

[1]The most sophisticated articulation of this argument is made by Aaron and Schwartz (1984); for a recent update, see Aaron and Schwartz (1990). Among those advancing arguments for age-based rationing are Callahan (1987) and Lamm (1987). For a description of Oregon's approach to rationing, see Fox and Leichter (1991) and Brown (1991); both reports appear in an issue of *Health Affairs* that focuses on Oregon's priority setting.

more. Medicine's untested and often conflicting theories of efficacy justi-fy—and the dominance of professional preferences ensures—the full de-ployment of resources, no matter how many or in what quantities. Indeed, medical theory is often implicit and closely associated with per-capita quan-tities of supply such as hospital beds and physician subspecialists. The crisis in costs is the inevitable consequence of the policies of growth that have prevailed in the U.S. health care sector: the open-ended financing of entitlement services based on funding of utilization; the accelerated produc-tion of manpower based on perceptions during the 1960s and 1970s of a "shortage" in medical manpower; the specialization of the physician work force and its division into technology-driven subspecialties whose work-loads have uncertain impacts on the health status and satisfaction of pa-tients; easy access to capital markets for the construction of facilities and the purchase of technology; and a willingness of payers to reimburse for services involving underevaluated technology. The end result of these pol-icies has been quantities of supply that are well in excess of the amount required to produce and deliver services that are known to work or that patients are known to want. Under this interpretation, policies of health care limits should concentrate on global restrictions on growth and the promotion of strategies to learn what works and what patients want.

As one familiar with the patterns of use of medical care and the strengths and weaknesses of the scientific status of clinical medicine, I find a good deal of evidence in favor of the supplier-induced theory of demand.[2] This paper seeks to explain this point of view in more detail. It examines alter-native interpretations of the shape of the benefit-utilization curve to raise the "which rate is right?" question; that is, what is the rate of service use (and the amount of resources required) when supplier-induced demand is reduced—when patients are informed of the state of medical progress (what is known and not known about the results of care) and when patients are free to choose according to their own preferences? It then looks at the struggle between two competing models for reforming the doctor-patient relationship. One is based on the assumption that the agency role of the physician can be essentially replaced by the guardianship of the third-party payer through micromanaged care and that the delegated decision model inherent in the agency role can be preserved by prescriptive rules of prac-tice developed by competing health care organizations or the state. The

---

[2]The theoretical basis of this argument was developed in Wennberg and colleagues (1982). Archie Cochrane's *Effectiveness and Efficiency* (1972) provides a thorough introduction to the problems of physicians in understanding the outcomes of care; Eddy and Billings (1988) provide a more recent example. Much of the epidemiological evidence concerning the prob-lem of supplier-induced demand is summarized in "Small Area Analysis and the Medical Care Outcome Problem" (Wennberg, 1990a).

other is based on replacing the delegated decision model with shared decision making, a new partnership between the patient and the physician and the profession and the public. The target in this approach is to reform the ethical status of the doctor-patient relationship so that what is known and not known are explicitly shared and so that patient preferences become dominant in the choice of treatment from among reasonable and available plans of care. The paper also examines why neither micromanaged care nor the shared decision model are sufficient to achieve the goal of rationalizing utilization and containing costs. The implicit nature of much of medical theory keeps most of clinical practice outside of their influences. The paper thus argues that to contain costs it is necessary to limit capacity directly, and it sets out several principles to guide debate about strategies for developing limits. The paper concludes with a discussion of the implications for innovation of policies of limits in medicine.

THE SHAPE OF MEDICINE'S BENEFIT-UTILIZATION CURVE

Different assumptions about the relationship between the utilization of care and the benefits of care are reflected in different assumptions about the shape of the benefit-utilization curve in medicine. The assumption that it is necessary to ration specific services that work and that patients want but that society cannot afford is based on two ideas. One is the notion of "expected value" or benefit now obtained from the resources invested in health care. The doctor-patient relationship efficiently distributes care in such a way that patients benefit from the care they now use more than they would if the care were not received or if it were replaced by a less costly item or service. The other idea is that the "marginal returns" can be rationalized; that is, the benefits are sufficiently well understood that they can be ranked in terms of expected benefit per unit of service (or dollars) utilized.

The diminishing marginal returns that occur in an economy in which utilization is the result of patient demand and biomedical progress are illustrated in Figure 2-1. To achieve such a curve, physicians must be remarkably successful in the sorting of medical problems and in diagnosing and ranking them according to the expected outcomes of treatments. Indeed, they must be perfect in the execution of their agency role to interpret clinical science and understand the values their patients assign to alternative treatments, including the value of no treatment at all. They must thus possess something that clinical science does not now provide: knowledge about the outcomes that matter to patients. The problem the physician faces, however, is not simply to know the outcomes but to weight them according to the individual patient's attitudes toward them. Under delegated decision making, which has been the dominant medical decision model

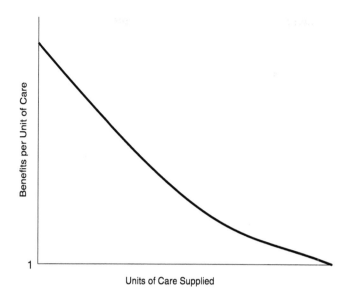

FIGURE 2-1   Example of benefit-utilization curve where medical progress and patient demand drive utilization with diminishing marginal returns.   The curve is
adapted from Aaron and Schwartz *The Painful Prescription: Rationing Hospital
Care*, p. 11.

since the time of Hippocrates,[3] physicians make the choices.   They intuit
what patients would choose if patients had full information about choices
and could do the weighting themselves.   In this model, prescriptions for
treatment are based on clinical experience, that is, on the "case series" of
patients that the individual physician has treated and whose values and
preferences have somehow become known.

At the level of the population, the situation is even more complex.   For
the curve to take its hypothesized shape of decreasing marginal social return, physicians must, collectively, make ordered choices; that is, the patient who receives the first unit of service is the one who gains the most
benefit from it, the second patient the one who gains the second most benefit, and so on, with the patient who receives the last unit gaining the least.
For this to occur, however, physicians must know and respond to decisions
their colleagues have made.   There is no feedback loop currently operating
in health care markets that would make this feasible; indeed, it is difficult
to conceive what such a mechanism would look like.

---

[3]See *The Silent World of Doctor and Patient* by Jay Katz (1984) for an excellent history of
the doctor-patient relationship.

Outcomes and preference research provide empirical evidence that demonstrates the weaknesses of the assumption that the benefit-utilization curves in medicine correspond to Figure 2-1. Over the past few years, my colleagues and I have been involved in an in-depth investigation of the fine structure of a clinical decision problem: the choices that face men with a common form of prostate disease called benign prostatic hyperplasia, or BPH. The inquiry was motivated by small area variation studies showing that the chances that a man would undergo a prostate operation by the time he reached age 85 varied from about 15 percent in some communities to more than 50 percent in others. We asked a group of Maine urologists, some of whom lived in areas with low rates, others of whom lived in high-rate communities, if they could explain these variations.

The urologists differed in their assumptions about the benefits to be derived from prostate operations and about the shape of the curve relating benefits to utilization. Some held a pessimistic attitude toward prostate disease. These physicians believed that BPH usually progressed to a life-threatening obstruction of the bladder or kidney and that it was best to operate early in the course of the disease to prevent future bad outcomes. We called this the preventive theory of surgery. Their clinical decisions were dominated by a hypothesized benefit-utilization curve in which the chief benefit of surgery was improvement in life expectancy. Their reasoning was that if surgery were postponed until evidence of life-threatening obstruction appeared, the patient would be older, sicker, and more likely to die when surgery finally became unavoidable. By operating early, one avoided the higher death rates that occurred when the operation was postponed. Because most men who exhibit early disease will progress to the point where surgery is inevitable, and because the death rate from surgery increases with age, BPH patients will live longer if they have the operation earlier. Because most men eventually develop BPH symptoms, the population captured under the benefit curve of preventive theory (Figure 2-2) encompasses the majority of older men.

Other urologists were more optimistic about untreated BPH and argued for the quality of life theory of surgery. This theory posits that the benefit of surgery for men without obstruction of the bladder or kidneys is its ability to reduce symptoms and improve the quality of life. In the opinion of these urologists, BPH does not usually progress to the point where it threatens life; accordingly, surgery does not play a preventive role in avoiding early death. They estimated that a patient's "utility" for surgery—that is, the "expected value" the patient would gain if the surgeon prescribed surgery—was greatest for those with severe symptoms, whereas those with mild symptoms benefited little. The benefit-utilization curve suggested by these physicians (Figure 2-3) thus has a different parameter of benefit as well as a more rapid decline in value.

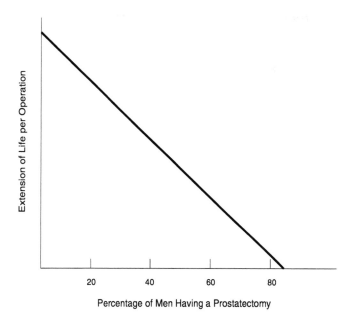

FIGURE 2-2   Benefit-utilization curve under the theory that prostate surgery increases life expectancy.

The unresolved competition between the preventive and the quality of life theories (and their corresponding benefit-utilization curves) reflects indeterminacy rooted in poor clinical science. The outcomes research we undertook showed that the preventive theory was incorrect.[4] Early surgery appeared to lead to a slight decrease in life expectancy because for most men BPH does not progress to life-threatening obstruction. Those without evidence of such obstruction were better off with watchful waiting if the expected value of treatment was an increase in life expectancy. The curve in Figure 2-2 thus is incorrect. If prostate surgery has a place for men with symptoms, it lies in accordance with the quality of life theory.

But the uncertainty about the shape of the benefit-utilization curve is more profound than the failure to define and measure the outcomes that matter to patients. Most urologists who believed in the quality of life hypothesis also practiced within the delegated decision tradition. They understood that they bore a responsibility as the patient's agent to interpret

---

[4]The findings of this research project have been widely reported. For examples, see Wennberg et al. (1988); Fowler et al. (1988); and Barry et al. (1988).

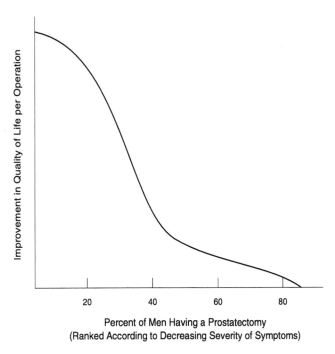

FIGURE 2-3   Benefit-utilization curve under the theory that prostate surgery improves quality of life.

for him what he needed and to convince him, for reasons of his own best interest, to accept their prescription. Yet our preference research showed that what patients want cannot be predicted from objective information available to the physician—that is, from data gained during the physical examination, from laboratory tests measuring such factors as urine flow, or even from answers to questions about the severity of symptoms or impairment of quality of life. Patients who by all such objective measures are similar may still differ in their preferences for treatment. Indeed, as it turned out, when they were informed about the alternatives and offered a choice, nearly 80 percent of men with severe symptoms choose watchful waiting, at least initially. Preferences for outcomes and level of aversion to risk cannot be intuited reliably by physicians based on objective knowledge; to know what patients want, physicians must ask them.

When patient preferences are neglected or misunderstood, the benefit-utilization curve is erratic, without evidence of rational sorting, and the net expected value can actually be negative. For example, if 16 severely symptomatic men were ranked according to impairment of urine flow (a common

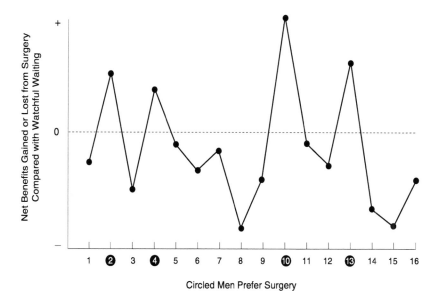

FIGURE 2-4 Benefit-utilization curve for 16 men with severe prostate symptoms who were prescribed surgery under the delegated decision making model.

diagnostic tool), our studies predict that only 4 would want surgery and that the 4 choosing surgery would not be correlated with urine flow impairment. If surgery were prescribed for all 16 men on the basis of the delegated decision model—that is, without informing patients about their options and asking them what they wanted—most patients would receive care they did not want. Whereas the patients ranked second, fourth, tenth, and thirteenth may want surgery, the majority do not. For these patients, the expected value of surgery is actually negative, compared with the benefit they would have obtained from the watchful waiting option they wanted (Figure 2-4).

WHICH RATE IS RIGHT?

What is the rate of service (and resource) use when patients are informed about the state of medical progress—about what is known and not known about the relationship between treatment options and the outcomes that matter to patients—and are free to choose among options according to their own preferences? What are their attitudes toward the benefits and risks of the expected outcomes?

Preference research gives a tentative answer. When patients with BPH are fully informed about their treatment options and asked to participate in clinical decisions, they choose less invasive treatments more often than they do when decision making follows the delegated model; their choice of treatment is strongly influenced by the degree to which they are bothered by their symptoms and their fear of impotence. Moreover, the population-based rates of surgery decline. For this condition, the trend toward conservative (nonsurgical) treatment choice is evident even in prepaid group practices in which the rates of surgery were already relatively low (and where patients faced no cost barriers at the point of delivery). The results of our preference research thus indicate the likelihood of significant negative returns on current patterns of resource deployment under the delegated decision model.

For the vast majority of illnesses and conditions, the pattern of variation in treatment choice is similar to or even greater than the variation seen for prostate disease. Most conditions do not have a single best treatment. For most conditions for which there is one or more "appropriate" surgical treatments there is also one or more nonsurgical options that are feasible within current scientific understanding. Surgical options for nine conditions—angina, arthritis of the hip and knee, silent gallstones, menopausal conditions affecting the uterus, peripheral vascular disease, back pain due to disc disease, atherosclerosis of the arteries of the neck, and BPH—account for well over half of the major surgery performed in the United States (Table 2-1). For these, the shape of the benefit-utilization curve is un-

TABLE 2-1 Common Conditions for Which the Shape of the Benefit-Utilization Curve Is Unknown

Condition	Major Treatment Controversies
Noncancerous condition of the uterus	Surgery (by type) vs. hormone treatment vs. drugs vs. watchful waiting
Angina pectoris	Bypass surgery vs. angioplasty vs. drugs
Gallstones	Surgery vs. stone crushing vs. medical management vs. watchful waiting
Peripheral vascular disease	Bypass surgery vs. angioplasty vs. medical management
Cataracts	Lens extraction (by type) vs. watchful waiting
Arthritis of hip and knee	Surgery (by type) vs. medical management
Prostatism (BPH—benign prostatic hyperplasia)	Surgery (by type) vs. balloon dilation vs. drugs vs. microwave diathermy vs. watchful waiting
Herniated disc	Surgery (by type) vs. various medical management strategies
Atherosclerosis of carotid artery with threat of stroke	Carotid endarterectomy vs. aspirin

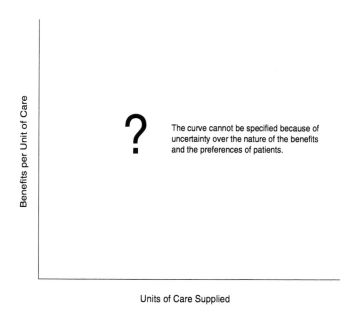

FIGURE 2-5   Status of the current understanding of the benefit-utilization relationship for most medical treatment theories.

known (see Figure 2-5). Through outcomes research, however, and the distinguishing of patient preferences from those of the physician, it will be possible to create islands of rationality in a sea of uncertainty and supplier-induced demand.

REFORM OF THE DOCTOR-PATIENT RELATIONSHIP

The flaws in the role of the physician as a decision-making agent for the patient are now widely apparent, and reform of the doctor-patient relationship is under way. The question now is, which model will replace it? In the United States, ambitious programs have been implemented to check the autonomy of the physician by imposing the use of clinical policy managers to micromanage the choices doctors make for their patients. Unlike the classic staff-model health maintenance organization (HMO) in which cost containment is achieved through global restrictions on the quantity of supply, the strategy of micromanaged care is to force efficiency by setting parameters of practice to define the available options and to guide a myriad of everyday clinical decisions. Acting as agents for third-party payers, the micromanagers develop rules of practice and use them to patrol the decisions of physicians. Virtually all major insurance companies offer micro-managed care programs that invade the traditional decision-making authority of physicians, subjecting their prescribing authority to the discipline of rules developed and administered by third parties. The strategy is not limited to private payers: the state of Oregon, while setting an overall budget, administers constraints not through global budgeting or overall limits on resources but through an ambitious program to micromanage benefits (services) based on estimates of relative cost-effectiveness.

This author's criticism of the micromanaged care model is based in part on its failure to understand the limitations of clinical science. The strategy assumes that the shape of the benefit-utilization curve is known and that this knowledge can be codified by the committees of experts convened to write the rules of practice. Inevitably, because of defects in the knowledge base of medicine which were discussed earlier, virtually none of the rules that emerge from this process can be based on an understanding of the structure of the decision problem over which they claim authority. Because the process is decentralized—there seem to be well over a hundred parties engaged in rule setting—the results are a plethora of varying prescriptive or advisory codifications of the rules of practice, some that directly conflict with one another. In an unfortunate number of examples, the rules are secret or proprietary, the property of the managed care company.

This critique is also based on the ethical weakness of micromanaged care—that is, its tendency to preserve the delegated decision-making model by substituting the guardianship of the third party for the benevolent authoritarianism of the physician. There is little pretense that this model of reform concerns itself with the preferences of individual patients. The imposition of third-party rule often occurs through telephone conversations over an 800 number involving the physician and the agent of the third party. Patients are not involved. The irony is obvious: if physicians do not know what works and what patients want, how can the third party claim such knowledge? The substitution, however, is not simply that of one imperfect agent for another. The micromanagers are agents of the payer, not the patient. The intrusion opens the doctor-patient relationship to the free play of various interests in setting and enforcing clinical rules, a circumstance that offers numerous opportunities for irrationally and arbitrarily rationing care and otherwise perverting the struggle to base clinical choice on the preferences of patients.

The opposing model for reform centers on what would be required to facilitate the sharing of decision making by patients and physicians. It depends on a program of outcomes and preference research and on philosophical inquiry to build the scientific and ethical base for helping patients make decisions that reflect their preferences. It depends on a new relationship between doctors and patients, based on open communication and the development of new styles of discourse and trust. Shared decision making competes for authority with micromanaged care. Each model seeks to influence clinical choice in specific nonemergency situations such as those listed in Table 2-1, situations in which options exist and time is available to reach a decision. Most commonly, these choices involve the elective use of surgery, but the participants in the conversation are different from those in the managed care model. There, the conversation takes place between the payer and the physician; in shared decision making, discourse is between the physician and the patient.

Because of its explicitly ethical basis, the shared decision-making model is preferable when fateful choices must be made between elective treatment options that entail differing risks and benefits. In these situations, rational choice depends on finding out what the patient wants. As noted earlier, preferences cannot be diagnosed by physical examination, laboratory tests, or questionnaires about symptoms or quality of life. A patient who meets the managed care criteria of eligibility based on these objective features of "appropriate care" may be prescribed a treatment he or she does not want. The benefit-utilization curves that result under micromanaged care look like those shown in Figures 2-4 and 2-5. It is doubtful that effective communication with a patient can occur over an 800 number, no matter how interested the micromanager may be in patient preferences. The shared decision-making model is therefore appropriate for choosing treatments for patients with such common conditions as angina, gallstones, uterine bleeding, benign hypertrophy of the prostate, cataracts, back pain caused by herniated discs, and arthritis of the hip.

LINKAGE BETWEEN THE SUPPLY OF RESOURCES AND MEDICINE'S IMPLICIT THEORIES OF EFFICACY

The critique of third-party micromanaged care presented here also rests on the likely futility of such an approach in effectively limiting undisciplined growth of the health care system. This is a weakness of the shared decision-making model as well. Neither approach is likely to produce systemwide containment of costs, which requires a macroeconomic policy; reforms targeted at the microeconomy of the doctor-patient relationship are insufficient tools for disciplining the macroeconomy. The reason is that most of medicine's resources are not used to execute discrete treatment options specified by well-developed medical discourse. Condition-treatment options such as those listed in Table 2-1 are the exception; most medical resources are allocated implicitly in varying patterns or cascades of acts undertaken to solve medical problems. The theoretical reasons for one pattern of allocation compared with another are often implicit and inaccessible to precise rules of practice. Indeed, medical theories are often so closely associated with the supply of medical resources that physicians do not even recognize them as explicit theories.

The effect of the supply of beds on the clinical thresholds for hospitalizing patients is a good example. The supply of hospital resources varies remarkably across geographic areas, and the amount allocated is unrelated to illness rates or to explicit theories about the numbers of beds required to treat most diseases. When more beds become available, they are allocated across a broad range of medical conditions for which the clinical policies governing admission and readmission rates are correlated with the supply of beds. In areas with fewer beds, patients with these conditions are more often treated outside of the hospital. For only a few medical conditions are the clinical thresholds such that illness rates determine the probability of hospitalization.

Let us consider the example of Boston, Massachusetts, and New Haven, Connecticut. Residents of Boston have about 4.5 hospital beds per 1,000 persons whereas New Havenites have only 2.9. Explicit rules of practice, codified in medical texts, dictate hospitalization for all patients with heart attacks or strokes, for those who need major surgery to treat their cancers, and for those who suffer from major trauma such as a hip fracture. Diagnostic criteria for these conditions are explicit, and the technologies for distinguishing the presence or absence of the condition are well advanced. But hospitalization for patients with these conditions requires less than 20 percent of the available medical beds, even in low-bed-rate areas. Most of the beds are used for conditions that exhibit highly variable patterns of admission. Hospitalizations for low back pain are the single most important reason for the difference in bed use between Boston and New Haven. Gastroenteritis is the second, followed by chronic bronchitis and pneumonia. The implicit rules of practice in Boston, which have been adapted to the greater supply of beds, result in a larger proportion of the population being admitted, with more frequent readmissions and shorter intervals between admissions.

The mechanism underneath the association between beds and admission and readmission thresholds centers on the decision making of physicians who must decide what to do with sick people. Imagine someone who is faced with the task of watching a conveyor belt that presents, in seemingly random order, a series of balls—some black, some white, some in varying shades of grey. The rules require that all black balls be picked up and put on a shelf and that white balls be left on the conveyor belt. The sorting task is to examine each of the grey balls and decide whether they should be put on the shelf—but at the same time to save room for all the black balls that must be put there.

The conveyor belt simulates the flow of patients through the emergency room or the doctor's office. The black balls are the conditions that all physicians agree require hospitalization; regardless of how sick the patient may appear, he or she must be admitted. The white balls are those conditions that are treated outside of the hospital. The task is to decide which grey balls should be "admitted"—placed on the shelf. Each must be evaluated as to its degree of greyness (relative illness). There are always more grey balls (more sick people) than there is room on the shelf. The sorter must find a way to deal with the problems presented by all of the grey balls.

Making judgments about degrees of illness and finding safe alternatives for patients are difficult tasks and involve a great deal of uncertainty. If beds are available, it is much easier to rely on others—the ward physicians and nurses—to sort out the problems. It is far easier to admit a patient to the hospital (put a grey ball on the shelf) than to search out alternatives.

Small area analysis reveals something that the sorters do not know. There are fewer beds per capita in New Haven; consequently, the shelf there is much smaller than the shelf in Boston—about half its size. In New Haven, the sorter must spend more time evaluating shades of grey and finding safe alternatives by making calls to the patient's private physician, eliciting the help of home health agencies, or arranging transportation to nursing homes, hospices, or departments of social services.

Small area studies reveal another curious feature: about the same amount of space on the shelf is held in reserve in the low-rate areas as in the high-rate ones. Despite the greatly reduced size of their shelves, there is no evidence that physicians in areas with low per-capita bed rates believe that they are rationing effective services. They do not even use all of the beds available to them. Clinicians in New Haven, like their counterparts in Boston, tend to hold about 15 percent of beds in reserve. They seem unaware of scarcity and are satisfied that their theories of how hospital resources should be deployed are appropriate. The chiefs of service at Yale's teaching hospital in New Haven, when asked whether they were aware that treatments were being withheld because of the area's per-capita bed supply, could identify no examples of explicit rationing. Indeed, as is so often the case when the facts of variation are presented, the chiefs were not even aware that hospital resources were relatively scarce in their community.

In the upside-down economy of medical care, supply comes first and theory follows, in virtual equilibrium as practice style adjusts to ensure the utilization of available resources. Thus, treatment theories governing the use of hospital beds are sufficiently flexible to allow the use of available beds, no matter what the per-capita level of supply; theories that establish the legitimacy of the use of particular procedures justify professional workloads, virtually without regard for the number of specialists; and underevaluated medical treatment theory is sufficiently rich to permit the employment of internists and family practitioners virtually without regard to how many there may be per capita. As clinical problem solvers, it is in the nature of physicians to deploy available resources, including themselves, close to the point of scarcity. They do this in pursuit of treatment theories that seem reasonable and that might just prove to be effective. This behavior is not the result of simple self-interest; it arises from physicians' perceptions of their role as healers, their faith in plausible theories of efficacy, and their willingness to work to find solutions to the endless stream of problems their patients present.

It is quite possible that higher per-capita rates of investment in health care produce no net benefit over what is achieved in areas with lower per-capita rates. Consider the evidence regarding bed supply. Much of the additional pool of resources in Boston is invested in more frequent readmissions of the chronically ill and in the care of terminal patients. In spite of the 70 percent greater per-capita expenditure for Bostonians compared with New Havenites, the mortality rates are the same, as predicted by the similarities in demographic characteristics. In addition, the more than twofold variation in expenditures for hospitalization among the 185 hospital service areas of New England is not correlated with mortality rates.

Indeed, why should greater spending bring better results? In formulating an expectation about whether more should be better, it is well to recall the contingencies that determine the capacity of the health care system. Capacity is not fashioned according to explicit theories about what works in medicine. The optimal number of beds is unknown, and the number that is actually built or supplied has no theoretical or empirical basis. (One looks in vain to medical texts to learn how many beds are needed for treating a population's burden of illness for such conditions as back pain, pneumonia, and gastroenteritis.) The number of beds is the result of the way the hospital industry has grown. Per-capita rates are arbitrary, the product of the opportunities and desires of institutions and communities—not of the needs or preferences of patients, shaped by the possibilities articulated by medical science.

This is easily seen in case studies that reveal the history of the planning and construction of hospital beds. The populations of Waterville and Augusta in Maine are about the same in size, but Waterville has nearly twice as many beds per capita. The reason is that Waterville hospitals were constructed according to the dictates of religious and professional orthodoxies, a set of dynamics that resulted in three hospitals: a Catholic and a Protestant hospital, each used by allopathic physicians, and a third hospital reserved for osteopaths. In Augusta, only one hospital was built, an ecumenical institution shared by all religious and professional persuasions. The medical care landscape in the United States is contoured by the jagged profiles of resource allocation exemplified by Boston, New Haven, Waterville, and Augusta. In each example, the intensity of construction is determined by dynamics that are indifferent to theories of efficacy or even to simple rules about the necessary numbers of beds in relation to the size of the population.

The number of physicians who are trained is governed by equally arbitrary policies, many of which were formulated in the 1960s, a period of great concern about medical scarcity. The number of physicians trained for each specialty is the product of administrative and political choices rather than a response to the resources required to produce services dictated by an answer to the "which rate is right?" question. In the case of procedure-oriented specialties, supply is well in excess of the number of practitioners needed to produce treatments that physicians agree are efficacious. For example, when neurosurgeons enter medical markets, they almost invariably find that the available supply has already taken care of the demand for surgical management of brain tumors and head trauma, which are the procedures that all physicians agree are needed. Neurosurgeons thus must invest most of their efforts in treating conditions for which there are valid nonsurgical options. The most common are two condition-treatment options listed in Table 2-1: back operations and carotid artery surgery. Although it is reasonable to conjecture that more of such surgeries might produce some benefit, the studies noted earlier suggest that the amount of neurosurgery now being supplied under the delegated decision model could well exceed the amount patients want when they choose according to well-informed preferences.

SEEKING LIMITS

It is quite possible that the current crisis in health care in this country may stem from the excesses of an economic sector dominated by supplier-induced demand and professional uncertainty about the value of medical care—and not from patient demand based on medical progress. The excesses arise because of errors in the assumption of neoclassic economic policy that capacity would be limited and the quality of care maintained by medical efficacy and patient demand, mediated through the physician who serves as the rational agent for patient and society. The effects of these errors are now increasingly apparent:

• *Quality is poor.* Patient values are not paramount in the decision to use care; information on options (and on the state of medical progress) is not freely communicated; and services (whether wanted or not) are produced with varying efficiency in regard to outcomes.

• *Costs are out of control.* The supplies of resources are created (in increasing amounts) without regard to explicit theories of efficacy and without knowledge of the shape of the benefit-utilization curves for medical interventions and of the amount of resources needed to produce the services patients want.

- *Access is diminished.* The decentralized structures that have financed care through insurance are increasingly unable to provide products that are affordable to business or to individuals without employment-based insurance.

It seems very likely that the 1990s will bring policy decisions that place explicit limits on the medical care system in the United States, although no model of governance has emerged as an odds-on favorite. It may well be impossible to reach a national consensus on what to do, in which case the initiative will fall to the states. If so, several models may evolve, but their shapes should be governed by certain principles and guidelines that find their empirical justification in the epidemiology of medical care and in ethics.

The first principle concerns the general welfare: *it is safe for patients and in the public interest to place global restrictions on growth in the capacity to provide medical care.* Studies of geographic variation in services in this country provide solid evidence that the capacity of the hospital industry and of the physician work force is now well in excess of that required to provide services that are efficacious and that patients actually want. Most medical resources are allocated to treatments for which the theoretical basis for allocation is implicitly associated with the supply of resources and for which there is no empirical evidence that more is better. The nation can and should deal directly with the forces of inflationary growth in the health care sector—with the policies that determine the numbers and distribution of manpower, the size of the hospital industry, and the quantities of technology. The excess in capacity means that the amount spent on health care (as a percentage of GNP) can be directly limited and a health care system achieved that is in equilibrium with other sectors of the national economy—without fear that valuable services must necessarily be rationed.

The second principle concerns the welfare of those who do not now have access to care because they lack insurance: *full entitlement of all Americans to health care can be instituted without increases in the proportion of GNP invested in health and without a loss of welfare to those now insured.* The fear that policies that extend health care entitlement to all citizens will exacerbate the cost crisis is unwarranted; the dynamics that determine the capacity and costs of health care markets are to a large extent independent of illness rates and the demands of patients. To see why this is so, let us return to the analogy of the person sorting the black, white, and grey balls. Physicians are unaware of the relative size of the resource shelf—that is, of the per-capita quantities of "supply" invested in their markets; put another way, they are unaware of the relative size of the population they are serving. For example, two-thirds of the population of Vermont could move to Boston before the relative size of the Boston hospital resource shelf approaches that of New Haven. The testimony of physicians in New Haven—and the statistical evidence that resources are held in reserve equally in all medical markets, regardless of the relative per-capita rate of resource investment—tells us that if the increase in population size occurred gradually, no one in the medical care industry serving Bostonians would notice the difference. The major change in practice style would be a change in the threshold for hospitalization—a more careful sorting of grey balls. The biggest change in the rates of use of hospitals would be for back pain, gastroenteritis, and chronic bronchitis.

Fewer than 15 percent of Americans are completely uninsured. An understanding of the epidemiology of medical care leads to the prediction that their entitlement would permit them to be absorbed into the health care system without loss of benefit to those now in the system and without any special increase in aggregate expenditures. The capacity to treat the uninsured is already there; what is needed is to make it possible for them to compete for the attention of the health care system on an equal basis with the insured. In a steady-state situation, the increases in costs for treating the uninsured will be offset by the savings realized by reducing utilization among those now insured.

The third principle concerns the interests of patients for whom expensive medical care is effective in a system characterized by excess capacity: *the resources required to meet unmet needs (e.g., prenatal care, bone marrow transplants, long-term care) should be obtained by reallocation of excess capacity and not by rationing effective care.* From the point of view of patients with costly diseases, the reallocation of excess capacity is a more humane way to meet unmet needs than is the deliberate withholding of expensive, effective care on the grounds that the benefits are too costly. If the people of Oregon decide that total resources for health care should be limited, then resources to meet unmet needs should be reallocated from areas of excess capacity. Oregon has its own Bostons and New Havens. Rather than withholding specific treatments such as bone marrow transplants, which are known to increase the expectation for life (and that patients are known to want), this principle recommends the reallocation of resources now invested in excess supplies of hospital beds. Large quantities of resources are thus available for reallocation. If the practice patterns of Boston were more like those of New Haven, 700 hospital beds would be unused, and in 1982 dollars, $300 million would be available for reallocation to other medical needs (Culp et al., 1987).

INNOVATION AND THE POLICIES OF LIMITS

Policies of limits that emphasize the rationing of care through prescriptive rules of practice, that is, through the micromanagement of the doctor-patient relationship, have very different implications for innovation than policies that set limits that have been developed in accordance with the principles set out in the previous section. The differences are key. At the level of the microeconomy—the doctor-patient relationship—the latter policies emphasize the underdevelopment of clinical science, the entanglement of preferences, and the implicit nature of much of medical theory. At the level of the macroeconomy, they emphasize the opportunities for meeting unmet needs that global limits and strategies for reallocating excess capacity open up. These opportunities also include the development of the necessary professional infrastructure to deal with the weaknesses in the scientific and ethical status of the doctor-patient relationship. A successful policy of global limits has the immediate consequence of buying time to learn what works in medicine and to sort out the many conflicting, explicit theories governing resource deployment in the treatment of discrete conditions such as those listed in Table 2-1. But the several European and the Canadian models for managing the macroeconomy show clearly that setting global limits does not of itself lead to improvement in clinical science or to the development of models for clinical decision making that emphasize patient preferences. For innovation along these lines to prosper, policies to achieve global limits must be linked to a science policy that builds the infrastructure for evaluating medical theory and promotes new models of the doctor-patient relationship.

The introduction suggests some of the characteristics of a science policy that would promote "rational" innovation under both policies of global limits and of managed care. Such policies would encourage the development of new ideas and technologies and their systematic evaluation in a context that fosters the progressive growth of a more fully rationalized microeconomy, namely, a doctor-patient relationship in which decisions are based on information about outcomes and on the preferences of patients. This chapter also draws attention to the sources of medical ideas and the current processes of evaluation to highlight the importance of problem solving in everyday practice as a source of medical theory. In addition, it emphasizes the lack of standardization in innovative processes when they occur in the context of the daily practice of medicine.

The varying sources of medical ideas and the complexity of the innovative processes of medicine have an important implication for science policy: evaluative research must be closely linked to daily practice. They also suggest two goals and two processes of evaluation:

1. the goal of theory evaluation, by which alternative treatments for common conditions are tested in a comprehensive, systematic approach; and

2. the goal of process evaluation, by which the various configurations for packaging technologies and organizing human resources and levels of skill are explicated and evaluated.

The first goal involves outcomes research, the second involves quality management, and their linkage is the relationship between their ends and the means for achieving them.

Let us briefly consider the requirements for building an infrastructure for the evaluative sciences in medicine. The first volume in this series discussed the various disciplines that constitute the evaluative sciences and the rationale for their introduction into mainstream thinking in medical schools (Wennberg, 1990b). It also discussed the policy basis for outcomes research and an organizational strategy, the patient outcome research team approach, for meeting the ongoing requirements for evaluation of established treatment theories, as well as innovations as they emerge. These teams—PORTs, as they are becoming known in the United States—are part of the infrastructure being developed by the Agency for Health Care Policy and Research, a new federal agency that represents the first explicit effort on the part of government to articulate science policy for the evaluative sciences.

There is a certain irony that public policy to rationalize health care should develop in the one nation among Western democracies that Brian Abel-Smith (1985) labels the "odd man out," the single example of a nation that has failed to establish policies of global limits on expenditures. The need for rational reallocation is most acute in systems of care in which marginal spending on innovation is inhibited by policies of global limits. Strategies for avoiding explicit health care rationing by reallocating excess capacity to meet unmet needs for effective medical care depends on the successes of the evaluative sciences in identifying examples of excess capacity and establishing evidence that care is, indeed, effective. It should be much easier to build the necessary infrastructure in systems of care in which the societal commitment to set limits is in place—once the problem of professional uncertainty and excess capacity is understood by policymakers. At least in principle, systems of care governed by policies that rationalize the deployment of manpower and budgets can redefine professional tasks much more easily than is now possible in the United States, with the important exception of prepaid staff-model HMOs such as the Kaiser Permanente Plan or Group Health Cooperative of Puget Sound.

The reallocation of professional time and talent toward the two goals of outcomes research and quality management is a clear example of a potential advantage that Canadian or European models have over the United States. For the sake of argument, let us assume that the health care industry, like any other high-technology industry, should allocate 10 percent of its earnings to the development and testing of its products. In the health care field, investments of this order of magnitude are now made only by well-capitalized pharmaceutical and medical device industries, and as the example of off-label uses of drugs such as prazosin shows, this does not lead to full rationalization of even drug-related clinical theory. The problem is the vast undercapitalization of the evaluative function within the ongoing practice of medicine. Resources to evaluate innovations arising in clinical practice or to undertake the quality management tasks that in most industries are part of the production process have not traditionally been made available by government or the private sector. One of the most constructive steps consistent with the principles outlined in the previous section would be to allocate a substantial proportion of the health care budget to the task of building the necessary professional infrastructure in the evaluative sciences.

Canada offers an example of what could be done in a system with global limits in place. Canadian physicians are currently paid much less on a per-procedure basis than their counterparts in the United States, resulting in longer work hours and greater productivity in terms of the numbers of procedures performed per physician; as a consequence, the rates of use of many common surgical procedures (and probably a good number of diagnostic procedures) in Canada rival those in the United States, even though the supply of specialists is considerably less. Some of the excess capacity that Canadians now allocate to such procedures could be safely allocated to conduct outcomes research and build the professional infrastructure for management of quality. Leading physicians who are interested in these tasks could be safely recruited from active practice without fear that the reduction in services would harm patients. (This could be done on a half-time basis to allow these physicians to remain clinically active.) Such an effort would not require a reorganization of the fee-for-service financial structure but only the willingness of the provincial government to negotiate salaries for physicians who chose to invest part of their professional time in this manner. Networks of recruited, professional talent linked to centers for the evaluative sciences, would form the infrastructure for a variety of evaluative tasks as well as the dissemination of results. Presumably, such a strategy would also be cost saving, because the total cost of care per active physician—the stream of medical acts he or she initiates or sustains—is very likely to be much greater than the total cost of research per physician-investigator. A commitment to evaluation along these lines holds the promise of rationalizing a spectrum of current inefficiencies, particularly in the management of quality and the explication of as yet unrecognized variations in the processes of production.

An all-payer or single-payer model also offers another opportunity for rapidly increasing the level of sophistication of practicing physicians in the evaluative sciences, in particular their understanding of the relevance of evaluation for the everyday practice of medicine. Medical education has been primarily geared to the production of medical students and the training of medical residents; in situations of perceived manpower scarcity, this focus is quite natural. The current situation of excess capacity presents a new challenge and opportunity for medical education: to pay attention to ongoing learning requirements in a field with rapid technological change and to commit to a mission of lifetime learning in which skills are reshaped, knowledge rebuilt, and careers refashioned to meet changing needs. Again, in Canada, these policies are within reach. Just as the existence of excess capacity justifies the redeployment of professional talent to build capacity for the evaluative sciences, it also justifies periodic salaried sabbaticals from clinical practice for all professionals, including physicians, nurses, administrators and others.

In theory, the British National Health Service provides similar flexibility for the reallocation of professional workloads. Moreover, the special role of the British general practitioner, the unique responsibility he or she bears for initiating referrals, offers a splendid opportunity for development of the new model for the doctor-patient relationship based on shared decision making. Rationalization of treatment patterns for specific conditions such as BPH ultimately depends on rationalization of referrals from primary care to specialty care—on the development of what in the United States is called the cognitive role of the physician.

It is no coincidence that governmental policy encouraging the evaluative sciences developed first in the United States. The issue of practice variations and the need to improve the scientific basis of clinical decision making have been prominently discussed in professional journals as well as in the lay press. The linkage of practice guidelines to outcomes research and the growth of the idea that micromanaged care will contain costs brought together the critical support needed for a new federal initiative, the Agency for Health Care Policy and Research, at a time of budget deficit and reluctance by Congress to take on new tasks. The tensions between the trend toward cost containment based on micromanaged care and the needs and requirements for rational innovation continue to grow. The implications of micromanaged care for the innovative processes of the pharmaceutical and medical device industry, as well as for surgical innovation, are now being widely discussed. In some cases, the emphasis on cost-effectiveness and reallocation will seem commensurate with the goals outlined here. But in other cases, the restrictions operate in the other direction and affect the weakest link in the evaluative process: the assessment of innovation within the context of everyday practice. At a time when the expansion of practice-based infrastructure to support innovation is needed, rules that restrict the funding of "experimental" technologies are being more rigidly enforced. Moreover, the increasing sensitivity to cost shifting, that is, the effort on the part of the purchaser to get the "right price," penalizes most the academic medical centers that traditionally have been the most productive sources of medical innovation. This is unfortunate, given that the health care system's situation of excess and professional uncertainty requires just the opposite.

Nevertheless, things are changing. Whatever the shape of the new American health care economy, the policies of reform, if they are to promote rather than retard medical innovation, must assume the obligation to build the scientific and ethical basis of clinical medicine and contain resource consumption within limits acceptable to the wider society. The obligation to reform the scientific and ethical basis of clinical medicine can be summarized in four guiding principles:

1. knowledge about relevant treatment options should be freely communicated to patients;
2. the choice of intervention from among options that work and that society is willing to provide should be based on the patient's preference;
3. the production of treatments should be continuously improved; and,
4. new as well as conventional treatment theories should be continuously assessed and reassessed.

The opportunity to build a productive microeconomy, to keep the doctor-patient relationship free from intrusions by the state or by third-party micromanagement, depends, in turn, on a public policy for health that deals with the problem of limits and innovation. The challenge to the policies and politics of reform is to (a) set limits on the growth of supply; (b) reallocate excess capacity to productive purposes; (c) support the lifetime learning requirements of the profession; and (d) build the professional infrastructure required to learn what works in medicine and to produce services efficiently, free of supplier-induced demand.

REFERENCES

Aaron, H. J., and Schwartz, W. B. 1984. *The Painful Prescription: Rationing Hospital Care.* Washington, D.C.: The Brookings Institution.

Aaron, H. J., and Schwartz, W. B. 1990. Rationing health care: The choice before us. *Science* 247:418-422.

Abel-Smith, B. 1985. Who is the odd man out: The experience of Western Europe in containing the costs of health care. *Milbank Memorial Fund Quarterly* 63:1-17.

Barry, M. J., Mulley, A. G. Jr., Fowler, F. J., and Wennberg, J. E. 1988. Watchful waiting vs. immediate transurethral resection for symptomatic prostatism: The importance of patients' preferences. *Journal of the American Medical Association* 259:3010-3017.

Brown, L. 1991. The national politics of Oregon's rationing plan. *Health Affairs* 10:28-51.

Callahan, D. 1987. *Setting Limits: Medical Goals in an Aging Society.* New York: Simon and Schuster.

Cochrane, A. 1972. *Effectiveness and Efficiency.* London: Nuffield Provincial Hospital Trust.

Culp, W. J., Freeman, J. L., and Wennberg, J. E. 1987. Are hospital services rationed in New Haven or overutilized in Boston? *Lancet* 1:1185-1188.

Eddy, D., and Billings, J. 1988. The quality of medical evidence: Implications for quality of care. *Health Affairs* 7:19-32.

Fowler, F. J., Wennberg, J. E., Timothy, R. P., et al. 1988. Symptom status and quality of life following prostatectomy. *Journal of the American Medical Association* 259:3018-3022.

Fox, D. M., and Leichter, H. M. 1991. Rationing care in Oregon: The new accountability. *Health Affairs* 10:7-27.

Katz, J. 1984. *The Silent World of Doctor and Patient.* New York: Free Press.

Lamm, R. D. 1987. Ethical care for the elderly. In: Smeeding, T. M., ed. *Should Medical Care Be Rationed by Age?* Totowa, N.J.: Rowman and Littlefield, pp. xi-xv.

Wennberg, J. E. 1990a. Small area analysis and the medical care outcome problem. In: AHCPR (Agency for Health Care Policy and Research) Conference Proceedings, *Research Methodology: Strengthening Causal Interpretations of Nonexperimental Data.* DHHS Pub. No. (PHS) 90-3454. Washington, D.C.: Department of Health and Human Services, pp. 177-206.

Wennberg, J. E. 1990b. What is outcomes research? In: A. C. Gelijns, ed. *Medical Innovation at the Crossroads.* Vol. 1, *Modern Methods of Clinical Investigation.* Washington, D.C.: National Academy Press, pp. 33-46.

Wennberg, J. E., Barnes, B., and Zubkoff, M. 1982. Professional uncertainty and the problem of supplier-induced demand. *Social Science and Medicine* 16:811-824.

Wennberg, J. E., Mulley, A. G. Jr., Hanley, D., Timothy, R. P., Fowler, F. J., Roos, N. P. Jr., et al. 1988. An assessment of prostatectomy for benign urinary tract obstruction. *Journal of the American Medical Association* 259:3027-3030.

Part II
Managing Care in the United States

3

The Growth of Managed Care
in the Private Sector

Michael Soper and David Ferriss

The private sector is moving rapidly into managed care.[1] Over the past two decades, profound changes have occurred in the way health care is organized and provided. The American health care delivery system has been transformed from one in which independent, fee-for-service medicine was dominant to one that is increasingly characterized by multiple health care delivery systems based on contractual relationships between managed care organizations and physician and institutional providers. This paper attempts to identify the factors responsible for this rapid movement toward managed care and to suggest consequences of this movement for the development and dissemination of medical technology.

EMPLOYER-PROVIDED HEALTH CARE BENEFITS
IN THE UNITED STATES

Employee group health insurance has been an accepted employer-provided benefit for some four decades in the United States (Feldman et al.,

[1] *Managed care*: A term often used generically for all types of integrated delivery systems, such as HMOs and preferred provider organizations, implying that they "manage" the care received by consumers (in contrast to traditional fee-for-service care, which is "unmanaged").

The terms defined in footnotes are based in part on a working paper by Jonathan P. Weiner and Gregory de Lissovoy of the Johns Hopkins University School of Hygiene and Public Health, Baltimore, Maryland.

1989). Since the end of World War II, an increasing number of employees and their dependents have been covered by group health insurance plans; in 1988, 153.3 million individuals were covered by some type of employer-related group health insurance (Health Insurance Association of America, 1990). These benefits traditionally have been provided through an indemnity insurance program; however, alternative systems of prepaid health care delivery have existed for some time (Mayer and Mayer, 1985).

Although employer-provided health care benefits have been of significant value to employees, the cost of providing these benefits has become increasingly burdensome to employers, particularly in an environment characterized by global competition. In a global marketplace, U.S. employers find themselves at a distinct competitive disadvantage because the high cost of health care—a cost of doing business in the United States—is not always a factor in the pricing schemes of competitors in other countries (Office of National Cost Estimates, 1990).

Even more alarming is the rapid rate at which health care costs have been increasing over the past two decades (Schieber, 1990). This rise is evident in the increasing proportion of the gross national product that is consumed by health care costs. A special concern of employers is that private-sector health care costs are inflating much more rapidly than those of the public sector, a fact that many employers and analysts attribute to cost shifting.

Cost shifting occurs when a health care provider, for example, a hospital, attempts to meet costs that are not fully covered by one purchaser of its services by "overcharging" other purchasers—in other words, shifting costs from one purchaser to another. To the extent that Medicare, as part of the Prospective Payment System, pays hospitals for services according to flat, diagnosis-related group (DRG) rates that do not cover a hospital's full costs for providing a service, the hospital must cover its unmet costs by increasing its charges to so-called passive payers—those payers who are not in a position to negotiate specific reimbursement amounts. Many argue that the private sector is being "taxed" (or overcharged) to support Medicare through this type of cost shifting. In a similar fashion, managed care organizations negotiate reimbursement contracts with hospitals and physicians, a course of action that effectively removes these organizations from the ranks of the passive payers. This strategy protects those employers who provide employee health care benefits through managed care organizations from further cost shifting, but it also results in a smaller number of passive payers onto whom providers can shift future costs. Traditionally, these passive payers have consisted primarily of indemnity health insurance companies.

Corporate America is quite serious about getting control of medical costs in order to stay in business; it considers itself literally in a fight for survival in an increasingly competitive global marketplace. This desire to contain medical costs is the major driving force behind the growth of managed care in the private sector. The next section of this paper examines those developments in managed care that have made this rapid growth possible. Prior to pursuing this theme, however, it is important to point out that managed care is not the only way to control health care benefit costs. Two other methods have been considered by employers: (1) relinquishing employer responsibility for the provision of employee health care benefits, and (2) sharing more of the costs of health care benefits with employees.

Relinquishing responsibility for the provision of employee health care benefits by transferring current benefit costs to increased salary and wages is attractive to many employers, because the inflation of salaries and wages is much less than that of benefit costs. The overwhelming majority of employers, however, realize that this approach is not a realistic option. Employer-paid health care benefits are firmly established in American society and are viewed as more of a right than a benefit by most employees. Given the current size of the U.S. deficit, it is unlikely that Congress will solve the significant health care access problems that presently exist by relieving American business of this responsibility. It is more likely that Congress will mandate some form of employer-financed health care benefits for those who are employed but who are currently without health care coverage, and extend public financing only to those who are unemployed.

The second method, sharing more of the costs of health care benefits with employees, has been extensively pursued by employers during the past decade. Although first-dollar, 100 percent coverage of health care costs by major employers was common in the past, it is rare today. This increased employee cost sharing has taken two forms: (1) employee contributions in the form of paycheck deductions and (2) the imposition of cost sharing at the time of receiving benefits.

Employees now tend to shoulder, through paycheck deductions, a higher proportion of the total premium cost of health insurance or its equivalent. This trend is particularly pronounced for the cost of dependent coverage. In addition, an increasing number of employers have introduced "cafeteria" benefit plans in which employees may choose what benefits they wish to purchase with a given number of employer-provided benefit dollars. Such plans are often an attempt by employers to help employees become more value-oriented purchasers of benefits, with hoped-for results that include increased awareness of the cost of employee benefits (in particular, health care benefits) and a decrease in the inflation rate of this cost.

In addition to increasing employee payroll deductions for health care benefits, employers have also sought to impose additional cost sharing at the time health care benefits are received. This most commonly takes the form of higher deductibles[2] and higher levels of coinsurance.[3] Deductibles of $200, $500, or more are now more the rule than the exception. To distribute the financial burden of higher deductibles more equitably, an increasing number of employers now set the deductible as a percentage of salary; thus, more highly compensated employees will pay a higher deductible before health care benefits apply than will lower paid employees.

A similar approach has been taken with coinsurance—the percentage of actual health care costs that an employee pays after the deductible has been met. Current coinsurance levels are typically 20 percent and in some instances may be higher. In addition, employers have increased the maximum out-of-pocket expense to which an employee is subject. Increasingly, this amount is also a percentage of the employee's salary rather than a fixed dollar amount.

The rationale for increasing employee out-of-pocket costs for health care services has been to give employees a significant personal incentive to consider carefully the costs as well as the benefits of these services. In increasing costs, employers would help their employees become more sophisticated, value-driven consumers of health care services. Without such incentives, employers would continue to bear the brunt of higher costs that arise, at least in part, from unrestricted use of the "health care credit card" by providers; employees (and providers) would continue to be the sole beneficiaries of the employer's largesse.

Although employers have pursued increased use of employee cost sharing for health care benefits, there are limits to the extent to which cost sharing can be imposed. High out-of-pocket costs may pose a significant barrier to access, thus inadvertently delaying needed treatment, which may result in poorer outcomes and higher health care costs. A second limitation comes from the intense dislike of employees for cost sharing and other "take-aways" from their health care benefits, a fact driven home by the willingness of organized labor to strike over this issue above all others.

Overall, the use of employee cost sharing to contain health care costs has not been successful. The "smart shopper" theory has proved to be flawed with respect to health care; sick patients have neither the inclination nor the information to shop around for the least costly health care option. Consequently, the amount of cost sharing that employers can impose on

---

[2]*Deductible*: That amount of covered medical care expense that the insured individual must pay before insurance benefits become effective (e.g., $200 per individual, $500 per family per year—a deductible may also be calculated on the basis of a percentage of an individual's annual income.)

[3]*Coinsurance*: That portion of the total covered medical expense paid by the insured individual after the deductible is met; coinsurance is usually expressed as a percentage of the total (e.g., 20 percent).

their employees has probably reached its limit, without appreciably slowing the health care inflation spiral.

An approach to containing health care costs by means other than increased employee cost sharing is to provide health care services through an alternative health care delivery system that attempts to give more value for the dollar in the form of lower costs and improved quality. In addition, its proponents hope that such an alternative system can favorably affect the rate at which health care costs are inflating. This is where managed care organizations enter the picture.

MANAGED CARE AND ITS GROWTH IN THE PRIVATE SECTOR

Managed care organizations do three things: (1) they establish a health care delivery system composed of physicians, hospitals, and other health care providers; (2) they merge the role of third-party payer with the role of provider; and (3) they actively manage the health care delivery process. In this way, managed care organizations both provide and manage health care, rather than just pay for it. They are active, not passive, players.

A major advantage of managed care organizations is that they significantly reduce the ability of providers to shift costs. Managed care organizations have contracts in place with both physician and institutional providers that specify and establish reimbursement arrangements. These arrangements are subject to negotiation and marketplace forces, but they constitute a real constraint on provider charges. In the private sector, other constraints on provider charges are few in number and weak in their effects.

For example, when health care is covered by passive payers, providers can increase their revenues by increasing the intensity (volume) of the service provided. Extensive diagnostic testing, prolonged hospital stays, and frequent follow-up visits are all examples of increased intensity of services for which the demand is strongly influenced by provider recommendations. The marginal benefit of such increased intensity is uncertain at best; fortunately, any potential harm or risk, if costs are not a consideration, seems even more remote. Given the lack of harm of such practices, little has been done until recently to interfere with the way providers manage the delivery of health care services. Indeed, the utilization management[4] practices of managed care companies that limit the delivery of some of these services are the only significant constraints in the private sector.

---

[4]*Utilization management*: The management of health resources so as to ensure that appropriate care is provided. Utilization management activities may include precertification of specific diagnostic and therapeutic procedures, authorization and concurrent review of inpatient treatment, management of catastrophic illness and injury cases, and discharge planning.

The more cost shifting that takes place, the greater the impetus for private-sector employers to move toward a managed care arrangement to avoid being the target of unrestricted increases in provider charges and intensity of services. This desire to avoid cost shifting is a significant impetus for the growth of managed care in the private sector; coupled with the desire of employers to eliminate inappropriate utilization of health care services, it has fueled an ever-increasing demand for managed care.

Changes have occurred in the managed care industry over the past 20 years to meet the demand of employers who want to move their employees into managed care delivery models. Such changes have been necessary to spur the development of a sufficient number of managed care organizations (all major health insurers now sponsor one or more) and more flexible products that encourage employees and their dependents to give up their historical freedom to choose their physicians and hospitals from among all of those available.

Although the concept of prepaid health care was well established prior to the 1970s, the Health Maintenance Organization Act of 1973 provided significant impetus to the health maintenance organization (HMO)[5] movement. The act was important in three respects: (1) it provided federal grants and loans for the development of new HMOs; (2) it superseded existing legislation in approximately 20 states, thus removing barriers to this type of health care delivery system; and (3) it provided an additional measure of credibility for HMOs as well as mandating employers to offer HMOs to their employees when HMOs were available (Soper et al., 1990).

---

[5]*Health maintenance organization* (HMO): A prepaid organized delivery system in which the organization and the primary care physicians assume some financial risk for the care provided to enrolled members. The term *health maintenance organization* was coined by Paul Ellwood for the Nixon administration in 1972. It constituted a renaming of two existing delivery models: prepaid group practices ("closed-panel" plans) and independent practice associations (IPAs, or "open-panel" plans). Currently there are four basic HMO models:

Staff-model HMO: A type of HMO in which the majority of enrollees are cared for by physicians who are on the "staff" of the HMO. Although these physicians may be involved in risk-sharing arrangements, a majority of their income is usually derived from a fixed salary.

Group-model HMO: A type of HMO in which a single large multispecialty group practice is the sole (or major) source of care for HMO enrollees.

Network-model HMO: A type of HMO in which a "network" of two or more existing group practices have contracted to care for the majority of patients enrolled in an HMO. A network-model HMO sometimes also contracts with individual providers in a fashion similar to the operation of an IPA-model HMO.

Independent practice association or IPA-model HMO: An "open-panel" type of HMO in which individual physicians (or small group practices) contract to provide care to enrolled members. The primary care physicians may be paid by capitation or by fees for service, often with a "withhold" risk-sharing provision. Physicians who participate in IPA-model HMOs retain their right to treat non-HMO patients on a fee-for-service basis.

In 1973, when the HMO Act was passed by Congress, only about 2 percent of private-sector employees were receiving their health care through HMOs. It was hoped that the new legislation would impel rapid growth of the HMO concept of comprehensive benefits and limited cost sharing within a cost-effective system of health care delivery. Despite high hopes, however, HMO growth during the 1970s was slow; other changes in the managed care model were necessary to bring about the eagerly anticipated growth of the concept.

One of these changes was a greater opportunity for developing independent practice association (IPA) HMOs. At the beginning of the 1970s, virtually all HMOs were of the staff- or group-model type. As these HMOs became successful and attracted increasing numbers of patients who were seeking more comprehensive benefits, physicians in private practice became concerned. The IPA-model HMO began to be viewed as a way for physicians to compete with the staff- and group-model HMOs without abandoning the private practice of medicine.

The development of IPA-model HMOs, which used the basic building blocks of mainstream medicine, allowed HMO growth to accelerate. This type of HMO avoided the problem of enormous cash outlays for building health care facilities and hiring physicians before sufficient members were enrolled. In the early 1980s, it became possible for for-profit companies to raise capital and invest in the development of IPA-model HMOs; this trend also facilitated the growth of the HMO movement.

As a result of these developments, most of the growth of HMOs in the 1980s came from IPA-model health plans rather than from staff- and group-model plans. IPA-model HMO enrollment increased from 19 percent of total HMO enrollment to 41 percent during 1980-1990. In 1985-1986 in particular, IPA-model HMOs surged in popularity, increasing from 181 to 345 (InterStudy, 1991).

The second important factor contributing to the rapid growth of managed care in the private sector has been the development of point-of-service (POS)[6] products, also referred to as open HMOs or open-ended HMOs. InterStudy, the Minneapolis-based HMO think tank founded by Paul Ellwood, characterizes these health care benefit products as follows: (1) people enroll in an HMO; (2) the HMO permits them to receive services outside of the HMO provider network without referral authorization but requires them to pay an additional deductible or a copayment, or both, to do so; (3)

---

[6]*Point-of-service (POS) plan* (also called an open-ended HMO or open HMO): A type of HMO in which the enrollees are not "locked in." Enrollees may leave the HMO and still have certain services covered. Such out-of-plan utilization is usually subject to a significant degree of cost sharing (e.g., deductibles and coinsurance) unlike those services delivered within the plan.

coverage is offered under a financing mechanism similar to traditional indemnity insurance and is available at any time service is desired; and (4) benefits for services received outside the HMO network are typically less comprehensive than the HMO benefit and usually include deductibles, co-payments, or coinsurance (InterStudy, 1991).

Behind the popularity of point-of-service products—popularity that extends both to employees and employers—is the fact that Americans like to have choices. Many Americans do not wish to give up entirely, in return for better benefits and lower out-of-pocket costs, the freedom to choose their own physicians and hospitals. The point-of-service product allows the employee to take advantage of the comprehensive benefit package and low out-of-pocket costs associated with HMO membership while retaining the right to seek care outside the HMO system from any licensed provider in return for higher deductibles and coinsurance. Employees can try the HMO, but if they find it not to their liking, they are not locked in to using it.

Point-of-service health care benefit products also have advantages for employers. Employers can offer their employees a single product that can operate either as a traditional HMO or as a traditional indemnity health insurance program. Employees who always use the HMO system receive all the benefits associated with membership in a traditional HMO; employees who ignore the HMO and consistently seek care from other providers still have indemnity benefits; and employees who use the plan in both ways have increased flexibility in meeting their health care needs.

Point-of-service products have also allowed employers with traditional indemnity programs to ease their employees into a more flexible managed care program without completely mandating that employees use only the HMO system of physician and hospital providers. The employer's hope, of course, is that employees will be attracted to HMO providers whose use ensures the most comprehensive benefits and least out-of-pocket cost. The benefits to the employer are better control of costs and an environment in which quality can be monitored and improved. As point-of-service products become more acceptable to employees, employers are likely to increase significantly the cost to employees of the opt-out component of such plans. Doing so will preserve freedom of choice but attach such a high price to it that receiving care outside the system will not be a realistic option for most employees in most cases.

Thus, the widespread development of IPA-model health plans and the availability of point-of-service products are facilitating the growth of managed care in the private sector, the implications of which are significant for the U.S. health care delivery system. As managed care becomes the dominant model for providing health care benefits, there will be fewer and fewer people to whom costs can be shifted, and cost shifting will come to an end. When no one is buying "retail" anymore, the "wholesale" price will have to be sufficient to cover the costs of providers of health care services. Less efficient providers that are unable to cover their costs will be forced to close. The most likely result will then be a far smaller number of more efficient, competing health care delivery systems rather than the thousands of independent physicians and dozens of redundant hospitals found today in most major urban areas. There will still be choices, but they will be fewer in number.

IMPLICATIONS OF MANAGED CARE FOR
TECHNOLOGY DEVELOPMENT AND DISSEMINATION

If, indeed, managed care continues to grow in the private sector, what are the implications of this growth for the development and dissemination of medical technology? The remainder of this paper addresses this question, particularly in the light of Wennberg's argument (in this volume) in support of global limits on health care resources as opposed to managed care.

In his paper, Wennberg argues for reform of the currently dominant delegated decision model in which the physician, without adequate knowledge of the shape of the benefit-utilization curve or the risk-benefit preferences of the patient, makes decisions regarding what patients need and want with respect to medical care. Wennberg advocates a shared decision model based on outcomes research and a sensitivity to the desires of the patient. He contrasts this model with managed care, a model, he argues, that concentrates on micromanaging physician decision making in the face of limited knowledge and without considering the desires of the patient. Both models, in Wennberg's assessment, are unlikely to control the continuing escalation in health care costs. To achieve this objective, Wennberg advocates a health care system that imposes global limits on the availability of health care resources. Such limits, he claims, will eliminate excess capacity (and therefore reduce costs) without compromising access to care that is medically appropriate and desired by patients. Wennberg cites studies of geographic variation in hospital utilization as evidence that physician and hospital bed supplies are in excess of what is required to provide care that is both effective and desired by patients.

Although it is true that managed care to a large extent has concentrated on reducing cost shifting, unnecessary hospital days, and inappropriate surgical procedures, it has also focused on improving the quality of medical care and the service that patients receive—that is, the outcomes of care, including patient satisfaction. This paper suggests that the managed care model has the greatest potential for bringing about both the transformation of the medical decision-making model and the appropriate allocation of health care resources that Wennberg advocates.

Managed care organizations, because they are systems, have the means to incorporate into physician practice behavior the results of patient outcomes research and the new technologies that support patient involvement in the medical decision-making process. As Wagner points out (in this volume), managed care organizations, in particular, HMOs, have a unique opportunity, with their defined populations and provider panels and their management information systems, to serve as valuable laboratories for research in patient outcomes, cost-effectiveness, and technology assessment. Rather than interfering with the physician-patient relationship, managed care organizations have the potential to enhance the relationship in a way that brings value to both parties, in terms of higher quality and satisfaction as well as reduced costs.

Wagner's example of how the Group Health Cooperative of Puget Sound, a staff-model HMO, made use of Wennberg's interactive computer video-disc technology to promote shared decision making between urologists and men with benign prostatic hyperplasia illustrates well the potential of managed care organizations to both improve the quality of medical care and contain costs. Although the incorporation of such technology in staff-model HMOs is more easily accomplished than in other types of managed care systems (e.g., IPA-model HMOs), there appear to be no absolute barriers to the incorporation of this kind of technology in less tightly structured managed care organizations.

With respect to excess physician and hospital bed capacity, it seems doubtful that the political will required to mandate resource ceilings will be found in the near future. In the past, certificate-of-need legislation has met with mixed success; the discipline of the marketplace may prove more acceptable to providers and consumers of health care services alike.

As the managed care sector continues to grow, an increasing volume of health care services will be provided through contracted provider systems—physicians, hospitals, ambulatory surgical centers, home health care agencies, laboratories, diagnostic imaging centers, and so on. Renewal of contracts by the managed care organization will increasingly depend on the ability of each provider to provide documented quality and service at a competitive price. In a competitive health care environment, providers who are unsuccessful at establishing themselves as high-quality, low-cost providers will have excess capacity and consequently will not survive. A reduction in excess medical care capacity will thus occur as the result of competitive rather than political forces.

The elimination of excess capacity in the managed care sector is further enhanced by the use of utilization management, procedures designed to assist the physician in determining which patients are the most appropriate candidates for a given clinical procedure and in identifying and coordinating alternatives to hospitalization. To use Wennberg's illustration of the black, white, and gray balls (see Chapter 2), managed care utilization management procedures have the potential to help physicians distinguish those patients—represented by the gray balls—for whom there is strong reason to believe that a given surgical procedure or course of inpatient care will be beneficial, from other patients—also represented by gray balls—who do not require a given surgical procedure or inpatient care and for whom other modalities or sites of treatment are more appropriate. The role of managed care is to help physicians avoid using excess capacity just because it exists. By resisting irrational demands for such services, managed care organizations alter the habits of physicians and hospitals that cause them to continue providing these services for no better reason than their availability. The effectiveness of utilization management is greatest for those cases (e.g., medical low back pain) that Wennberg identifies as showing wide, capacity-dependent variation.

A significant barrier to this approach, as Wennberg points out, has been inadequate knowledge of the benefit-utilization curve for specific clinical procedures; this is not a failure of managed care but simply inadequacy of collective clinical knowledge regarding the benefit of certain procedures and treatment modalities. Future advances in the study of patient outcomes, including functional health status and shared physician-patient decision making, will make it possible to develop utilization management procedures that are more scientifically based and that are oriented toward a physician education role rather than a policing mechanism.

In the opinion of these authors, the impact of managed care on the development and dissemination of technology is significant. A primary fact is that technologies that provide both demonstrated benefit to the patient and reduction of costs will be readily adopted by managed care organizations and readily disseminated through the health care system as increasing numbers of individuals are covered by managed health care arrangements. Technologies that are expensive and that have marginal or unproven benefit will be resisted by managed care organizations. The result will be increased pressure on the developers of a technology to demonstrate its benefit and its superiority over existing technology. Although the reluctance of managed care organizations to adopt a new technology before patient benefit has been clearly demonstrated may slow the process of new technology adoption and dissemination in the future, the longer-term benefit will be a more appropriate use of health care resources and additional assurance to the patient that a technology will be beneficial. The authors view this end result as a positive effect of managed care on technology development and dissemination.

Griner, in a companion paper (in this volume), discusses the notion of "hidden technologies," those new applications and enhancements of a new technology that develop as a result of daily application in clinical settings following the technology's introduction. Such innovation is a natural, and sometimes desirable, consequence of adoption and dissemination; however, uncontrolled innovation is not always beneficial to patients and often serves only to increase costs without increasing benefits. In some cases, the innovation may even prove to be detrimental to the patient. Within traditional indemnity health insurance mechanisms, these hidden technologies are difficult to recognize and control; with utilization management, managed care is able to resist their rapid adoption and to assess and introduce them in a more controlled manner, eventually adopting those that can be shown to provide increased patient value and rejecting those that do not.

The manner in which managed care organizations currently evaluate new technology—medical devices, pharmaceuticals and biologicals, and procedures—varies considerably from organization to organization. Small managed care organizations may have minimal or no internal capability for evaluating new technology; consequently, they rely on external sources of technology assessment. Large managed care organizations, particularly the national organizations, may have extensive internal resources for assessing new technologies and for making associated reimbursement decisions. Reimbursement for a given technology may vary from organization to organization, but it appears that managed care organizations will attempt to base their decision of whether to adopt a given technology not on the basis of its potential to increase their market share but on a careful review of empirical data from methodologically sound evaluative studies. In essence, managed care organizations will attempt to base their technology adoption decisions (and thus reimbursement) on the true benefit (or lack of benefit) of a technology. The scientific knowledge to support these decisions will not be sought or held for proprietary purposes.

Because of the complexity of the task of assessing new technologies, there is considerable interest in the United States in exploring ways in which managed care organizations, as well as traditional health insurers, might collectively support a level of technology assessment that is of higher quality than that currently possible for an individual organization to accomplish. Representatives of four managed care and indemnity health insurance company trade associations are currently exploring a public-private solution to the problem of valid technology assessment. Achieving such a mechanism, within the limitations of antitrust legislation, has the potential to facilitate technology assessment that is in the best interest of the public and that will continue to encourage appropriate technological development and dissemination.

Historically, managed care organizations and indemnity insurers have refused to pay for investigative or experimental technologies, arguing that funding such research is an appropriate role for government or private foundations and not for purchasers of health care benefits. This attitude, however, has been increasingly challenged by both medical research institutions and by patients seeking coverage for investigative treatments in the absence of effective conventional therapies (Newcomer, 1990). Largely as a result of increasing numbers of legal challenges to the policy of excluding investigative and experimental technologies from health insurance benefits, a number of managed care organizations and indemnity insurers have made exceptions to their existing policies of denying coverage for unproven technologies. In addition, U.S. Healthcare, a large regional HMO, and the Blue Cross/Blue Shield Association have announced their intent to support randomized clinical trials for evaluating the benefit of autologous bone marrow transplantation (ABMT) for women with breast cancer.

These authors believe that managed care organizations, in conjunction with traditional health care insurers, will be willing to support the evaluation of investigative and experimental technologies if uniform research protocols are employed across multiple sites. Adherence to uniform protocols would allow collection of sufficient patient data to allow statistically significant conclusions to be drawn. Currently, there is little uniformity, with the result that conclusions regarding the value of a given technology are delayed and difficult. Such a practice serves only to confuse the evaluation of new technology and does a disservice to patients, for whose care a technology may be used that ultimately proves to be without benefit or even harmful.

This paper concludes with several recommendations to help facilitate the development and dissemination of new technology within the dominant managed care environment of the future.

1. Managed care organizations should actively support outcomes research by making their data bases available to researchers in academic institutions and by participating in well-designed studies.

2. Managed care organizations should support the evaluation of selected new technologies when studies are performed using uniform, methodologically sound protocols.

3. Managed care organizations should refrain from competing for new technology on the basis of proprietary medical knowledge or exclusive coverage and instead should work cooperatively with the public sector to advance the state of medical knowledge and valid technology assessment.

4. Managed care organizations, with their defined populations and provider networks, should take advantage of their potential for ongoing health services research in the areas of patient outcome measurement, shared physician-patient decision making, and evaluation of new therapies, and should freely disseminate the knowledge that results from such research.

REFERENCES

Feldman, R., Dowd, B., Finch, M., and Cassou, S. 1989. *Employer-Based Health Insurance.* DHHS Pub. No. (PHS) 89-3434. Washington, D.C.: U.S. Department of Health and Human Services.

Health Insurance Association of America. 1990. *Source Book of Health Insurance Data: 1990.* Washington, D.C.: The Association, p. 7.

InterStudy. 1991. *The InterStudy Edge: Managed Care—A Decade in Review, 1980-1990.* Excelsior, Minn.: InterStudy.

Mayer, T. R., and Mayer, G. G. 1985. HMOs: Origins and development. *New England Journal of Medicine* 312:590-594.

Newcomer, L. N. 1990. Defining experimental therapy—a third-party payer's dilemma. *New England Journal of Medicine* 323:1702-1704.

Office of National Cost Estimates. 1990. National health expenditures, 1988. *Health Care Finance Review* 11(4):1-41.

Schieber, G. J. 1990. Health expenditures in major industrialized countries, 1960-87. *Health Care Finance Review* 11(4):159-167.

Soper, M. R., Stallmeyer, J. M., Bopp, K. D., and Wood, M. B. 1990. The HMO Act of 1973. In: E. J. Belzer, ed. *Balancing the Triad: Cost Containment, Quality of Service, and Quality of Care in Managed Care Systems.* Kansas City, Kan.: National Center for Managed Health Care Administration, pp. 12-18.

4

Managing Medical Practice: The Potential of HMOs

Edward H. Wagner

The traditional health maintenance organization (HMO), as defined by Donabedian (1983), remains an attractive paradigm for the provision of cost-effective health care. Prepayment imposes the discipline of a fixed budget, and responsibility for the full complement of services ensures a degree of balance between primary and specialty care. The presence of a defined population whose members have specific sources of primary care clarifies accountability, which permits epidemiologically based planning and management of primary and preventive care services. The successes of this model in reducing costs and hospitalizations without jeopardizing health status are reasonably well documented (Luft, 1981; Manning et al., 1984; Wagner and Bledsoe, 1990). Interestingly, these successes were evident in traditional HMOs like the Group Health Cooperative of Puget Sound (GHC) long before the formal management of care (e.g., guidelines or preadmission review) was in place. Strong, medically conservative cultures and the limitation of supply through controlled staff and bed expansion, analogous to the setting of global limits described by Wennberg (in this volume), would appear to be likely explanations.

However, in the previous chapter, Soper and Ferriss point out that traditional staff- and group-model HMOs have played only a small role in the recent rapid growth of capitated, managed health care systems. The new breed of HMOs are an array of acronymic insurance/delivery arrangements (Welch et al., 1990) characterized by capitation of some portion, often a small one, of a physician's practice. Many modern HMOs are little more than financial arrangements without the culture and resources associated with truly shared responsibility by provider and insurer for the full spectrum of services. In such organizations, managing care tends to rely on the "micromanagement" described by Wennberg.

There is another approach to managing medical practice besides the imposition of rules or restraints on provider decision making (micromanagement) or the restricting of capacity by setting global limits (macromanagement). This approach to managing care refers to a collaborative process for planning and delivering health services to a population. Its objectives are to optimize health status and satisfaction with care and to do so at a reasonable cost and with acceptable provider satisfaction. Well-managed care includes active efforts to ensure that cost-effective services are received, rather than only intervening to reduce or eliminate ineffective ones. Care management, from this perspective, focuses on the needs, preferences, and outcomes of subpopulations of consumers categorized by age, condition, or other relevant characteristics. Micromanaging care at the level of the individual patient through guidelines, reminders, or precertification review is part of this perspective, but perhaps not the major part. A population perspective forces attention to issues of supply, deployment of resources, and the organization of practice as well as "guidance" for individual patient decisions. It suggests an array of new intervention possibilities, such as the use of centralized resources for consumer and provider education, surveys of outcomes or preferences, and computer systems to create practice environments more conducive to providing cost-effective care (Wagner and Thompson, 1988).

Managing care to maximize outcomes requires collaboration among generalists, specialists, consumers, administrators, and evaluation scientists. Collaboration is facilitated by a strong provider organization and culture that is willing to consider other issues besides professional autonomy and reimbursement. Organized consumer involvement provides a clearer role and voice for patients. A balance among these perspectives is usually healthy and nourishes the roles of science and data as adjudicators of differences. Finally, managing care has often been a piecemeal operation—a little quality improvement here, utilization review there, a guideline here, and so forth. Paul Ellwood (1988) has urged that health plans develop "central nervous systems" to coordinate the various sensory and motor subsystems that influence outcomes. Traditional HMOs have many of these elements in place to varying degrees, but uncoordinated and uneven use of them limits the ability of managed care to improve outcomes or reduce cost inflation.

MANAGING CARE AT GHC

The way in which new technologies are handled at GHC, and by most group- or staff-model HMOs, illustrates both the problems and the potential of traditional HMOs (Figure 4-1). If a new idea surfaces, be it a preventive strategy, a drug, a device, or a significant change in protocol, it is referred to one of four standing committees: Prevention, Pharmacy and Therapeutics, Emerging Technologies, or Practice Efficacy (Guidelines). The most common sources of new ideas are GHC medical specialists who may be responding to a perceived community standard among their peers, to the clinical literature, or to the entreaties of a manufacturer. The committees, with varying degrees of clinical epidemiologic sophistication, review the literature and whatever local data might be available. An attractive, but expensive, new idea would require further review by management and governance structures responsible for coverage decisions. Ideally, implementation would be followed by evaluation and reassessment, but all too often this has not been the case.

The economic framework within which HMOs consider new technologies is outlined in Figure 4-2. The rectangle represents the HMO's budget, which is largely fixed by its various capitation arrangements. Price compe-

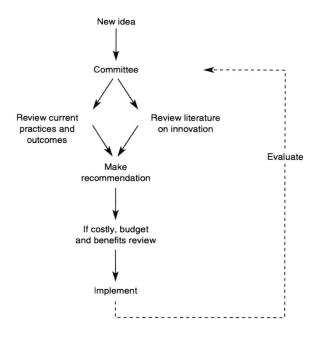

FIGURE 4-1 Clinical innovation management in HMOs.

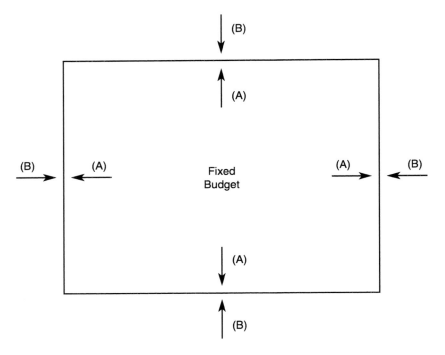

Arrows represent market forces:
(A) = New Technologies/Quality of Care Concerns
(B) = Price Competition/Lower Dues

FIGURE 4-2   Economics of innovation in an HMO.

tition, a reality of the past decade, presses inward. New technologies, presumably to improve quality of care, push outward because most will be covered by the comprehensive benefit.

BREAST CANCER SCREENING

The development and implementation of an organized breast cancer screening program illustrate the process and logic of innovation management at GHC. In fairness, this example shows the HMO at its best. The process began in 1982, although the first organized services were not delivered until 1985, which suggests both the deliberateness of the process and the difficulties of decision making in large organizations. In 1982, GHC had no formal breast cancer screening program, but rising demand was overloading available mammography units. Fewer than 10 percent of the 110,000 adult women patients of the HMO had had a GHC mammogram.

Data from the Western Washington Cancer Surveillance System (CSS) showed that the incidence of breast cancer among GHC women and the distribution of their stages of disease at diagnosis had been stable for 20 years. These data confirmed that minimal effective screening was taking place.

Growing provider and consumer pressure and an increasingly supportive literature convinced GHC's prevention leaders that it was time for the Committee on Prevention (COP; Thompson et al., 1989) to review the issue. The COP reviews possible preventive interventions using explicit criteria based on the World Health Organization criteria for screening (Wilson and Junger, 1968): the disease or risk factor must be important, detectable, and responsive to treatment, and treatment must reduce morbidity and mortality. The COP criteria also explicitly include consideration of the feasibility of implementation at GHC and the costs relative to other competing budget demands.

The COP appointed a breast cancer screening subcommittee of primary care physicians, epidemiologists, surgeons, radiologists, nurses, and health educators. In its addressing of the issue, the COP took a limited, budgetary perspective in assessing the economic impacts of various screening options on the HMO; in this instance, it attempted to estimate the costs of the additional screening associated with various screening program alternatives and the cost of evaluating those women with positive screening tests. Potential savings could occur if early-stage patients lived and paid dues longer, and required less costly care. Carter and colleagues (1987) identified all GHC women diagnosed with breast cancer in 1972 and gathered cost data on all diagnostic and treatment services they received for breast cancer over the ensuing decade or until death. Care for women with earlier-stage disease cost the system approximately $8,000 less than care for women with more advanced cancers.

The prevailing screening guidelines in the community at the time were those of the American Cancer Society (ACS), which recommended baseline mammography and a clinical exam at age 35, with annual screening beginning at age 50. In addition to their earlier analyses, Carter and coworkers (1987) also estimated the future costs to GHC, over the next 5 years, of either doing nothing differently or of implementing the ACS recommendations. According to their estimates, maintaining the status quo would not have generated sufficient screening activity to change the stage at diagnosis or the survival of many women, so it saved no money; on the cost side, it would require another mammography unit (at a cost of $231,000) simply to keep up with current demand. By contrast, implementation of the ACS guidelines would have substantially shifted the stage at diagnosis to earlier stages, added about 150 long-term survivors, and saved $2.6 million in breast cancer treatment costs and preserved dues revenues. Compliance with ACS guidelines, however, would have required new costs to the sys-

TABLE 4-1 Risk Factor–Based Screening for Breast Cancer

Risk Category	Risk Factors		Screening Interval	
	Women 40-49	Women 50+	Women 40-49	Women 50+
Level 1	Prior breast cancer, atypia, 2+ first-degree relatives	Same	Annually	Annually
Level 2	One first-degree relative	One first-degree relative or 2+ minor risk factors[a]	Every 2 years	Every 2 years
Level 3	At least one minor risk factor[a]	All other women	Every 3 years	Every 3 years
Level 4	All other women	Not applicable	On referral	Not applicable

[a]Minor risk factors include other family history of cancer, early menarche, late menopause, first birth after age 30 or nulliparity, or previous biopsy for benign disease.

tem estimated at $6.8 million. The net cost to GHC exceeded both $4 million and the realm of possibility.

In reviewing the breast cancer screening literature, the COP noted two points of interest:

• Conventional risk factors for breast cancer could be used to stratify women into subgroups with very different levels of risks (see Table 4-1), level 1 having 4 to 14 times the risk of level 4 (Carter et al., 1987; Taplin et al., 1990).

• The Swedish mammography trial (Tabar et al., 1985) screened women every 2 to 3 years, rather than annually, and achieved reductions in mortality comparable to that achieved by the annual screening evaluated in the Health Insurance Plan randomized trial (Shapiro et al., 1985).

These observations suggested the possibility of a risk-based approach to screening. The COP considered a program in which a computer-scored risk factor questionnaire would establish a woman's level of risk, which would determine the interval between visits to a centralized screening center (Table 4-1). At the center, women would receive a clinical breast examination by a trained nurse-practitioner, a mammogram, and instruction in breast self-examination. Questionnaires and invitations to the screening center would be sent directly to women by the program rather than by physician referral. Primary care physicians would provide annual clinical breast exams and reinforce the centralized program. Cost estimates, using the same methods as before, suggested shifts in the stage of disease at diagnosis and survival similar to the ACS approach, with the addition of women in their forties offsetting the losses associated with widened intervals between exams. Again, savings were estimated to be somewhat less than $3 million, but the estimated costs of screening were about the same (Carter et al., 1987). This hypothetical zero net cost proved to be a crucial selling point despite a startup cost of more than $1 million.

The COP sought approval but found no clear route. After a lengthy round of presentations to surgeons and radiologists, who feared patient overload; to primary care physicians, who feared loss of control; and to administrators, who were concerned about the budget, the Cooperative's Consumer Board of Trustees, led by its women members, finally approved the program and budget.

The program, now in its sixth year, has steadily increased the proportion of women having at least one GHC mammogram (Figure 4-3). Recent analyses of data from the Cancer Surveillance System suggest that the program has reduced the incidence of large and more advanced tumors among GHC women. Unlike other planned changes in medical practice, the Breast Cancer Screening Program is managed by a permanent steering committee and receives intense ongoing evaluation, supported in part by grant funds.

The GHC breast cancer screening experience illustrates both the wis-

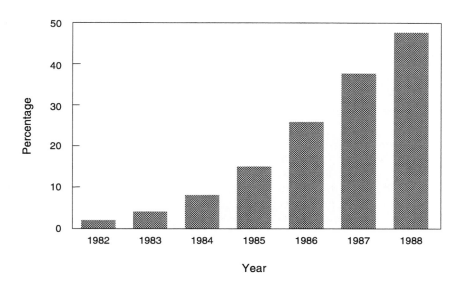

FIGURE 4-3   Percent of GHC women with GHC mammogram.

dom of and difficulties with this approach to managing care. The intensive use of trained epidemiologists and explicit criteria helped build a defensible case for a creative program, which has been systematically reported in the peer-reviewed literature (Carter et al., 1987; Taplin et al., 1990). Unfortunately, only the COP, of the four GHC committees, has that kind of evaluative science support. Formal, if limited, cost-outcome analysis was also essential to acceptance, and local data greatly strengthened the case. These analyses required laborious chart reviews, which could now be avoided by using computerized utilization and cost information. Consumer collaboration earlier in the process might have improved aspects of program design and increased program support as it went through budget deliberations. The major reason for the long development and decision process, however, was the absence of an organizational "central nervous system" with authority and accountability for changing medical practice. Instead, program developers faced what became a trip through Wonderland to get action on their ideas.

THE HMO AS EFFECTIVENESS LABORATORY

In the case of breast cancer screening, published randomized trials supported program development, but often this is not the case. In these latter situations, traditional HMOs have another opportunity—perhaps an obligation—to contribute more broadly to the effectiveness of medical practice by serving as laboratories for examinations of effectiveness and cost. All too often, careful review of the literature and available data do not support a clear recommendation about a new technology. The usual alternative is to leave it to clinical judgment, which, for new technologies, often means steady growth in use despite lack of formal review and approval. A second, better alternative is to conduct or participate in a formal study of a promising new idea and to coordinate the study with the HMO's decision-making process for the issue in question.

The randomized, controlled clinical trial (RCT) is the most persuasive basis for changing medical practice, a view now shared by practitioners as well as academicians. But the pace of progress by RCT is slow because of the constraints inherent in their use to answer urgent clinical questions. Given the manifold unanswered questions in clinical medicine and the generally high cost of classic, academically based clinical trials, more expeditious, cost-efficient mechanisms are needed for mounting RCTs to evaluate the costs and benefits of new technologies. Health care systems, especially HMOs, offer important and underdeveloped research resources.

Why should HMOs engage in the expensive, time-consuming, and, for most, very different business of conducting cost-effectiveness RCTs? Until recently, HMOs were far more interested in marketing surveys or evaluations of coverage changes and were reluctant to involve themselves in the complexities of studying care delivery. Now, however, health systems need to manage care delivery, and this requires the same kinds of evidence as are sought by the Health Care Financing Administration and the Agency for Health Care Policy and Research to meet national health policy objectives. Furthermore, managed care providers like HMOs now have information systems, patient populations, and research resources to gather the evidence for themselves. This creates an intriguing opportunity to accelerate the pace and relevance of outcomes or effectiveness research by encouraging research-oriented health systems to establish scientifically sound, locally relevant investigative activities to meet their own information needs as well as contribute to medical progress.

How this kind of research scenario might work can be illustrated briefly with the interactive computer videodisc, a technology developed by John Wennberg and his colleagues to facilitate shared decision making. The Wennberg team sought GHC interest in serving as a pilot site for the benign prostatic hyperplasia (BPH) interactive program (Selikowitz et al., 1990). GHC had no formal guidelines or review process for treatment of BPH; consequently, the HMO consulted its Committee on Practice Efficacy, GHC urologists, primary care leaders, and patient educators while deciding whether to participate in a pilot study. After further exposure to the idea and to a prototype, all agreed to the organization's participation in a pilot study, which was initiated in one of three GHC regions in November 1989.

Initial physician and patient response have been very positive. Age-adjusted rates of prostatectomy for each of GHC's three regions before and after the initiation of the pilot were calculated using the HMO's computerized data systems. Rates dropped in the pilot region shortly after the initiation of the program and have remained stable in the other two regions. These differences persisted throughout 1990. The positive pilot experience provided the basis for a more formal test of the program. Under the leadership of Michael Barry at Massachusetts General Hospital, federal funding was obtained to conduct a formal RCT of the approach in GHC's other two regions. The objectives of this experiment are to compare the shared decision-making program with a course of usual care, with respect to patient health and well-being, knowledge of their illness, willingness to participate in treatment decisions, and decisions that are finally made.

CONCLUSION

In the health care marketplace, the impact of the shift toward capitated and managed care on health care quality and costs remains uncertain. The heterogeneity of capitated arrangements and approaches to care management contributes to this uncertainty; it also militates against the opportunity

TABLE 4-2   System Characteristics of Health Maintenance Organizations Supportive of Managing Care

1. Defined population
2. Clear primary care accountability
3. Balance of power between primary and specialty care
4. Strong provider organization and culture
5. Organized consumer input
6. Access to scientific expertise and data
7. Structures and policies that limit capacity
8. Resources to support changes in practice style
9. Coordinated approach—"central nervous system"

of capitated, managed care to improve care and reduce costs, particularly if attention is not directed toward identifying those aspects of managed health systems that are important to improving outcomes and reducing costs (Ellwood, 1988). Table 4-2 suggests elements of HMOs that may be important for epidemiologically based management of care and for improving cost-effectiveness. Traditional staff- and group-model HMOs have many of these elements in place and remain important models for managing and researching medical practice, even if their potential in this area is still unrealized.

REFERENCES

Carter, A. P., Thompson, R. S., Bourdeau, R. V., et al. 1987. A clinically effective breast cancer screening program can be cost-effective, too. *Preventive Medicine* 16:19-34.

Donabedian, A. 1983. The quality of care in a health maintenance organization: A personal view. *Inquiry* 20:218-222.

Ellwood, P. M. 1988. Shattuck Lecture. Outcomes management: A technology of patient experience. *New England Journal of Medicine* 318:1549-1556.

Luft, H. S. 1981. *Health Maintenance Organizations: Dimensions of Performance.* New York: John Wiley, pp. 185-207.

Manning, W. G., Leibowitz, A., Goldberg, G. A., et al. 1984. A controlled trial of the effect of a prepaid group practice on use of services. *New England Journal of Medicine* 310:1505-1510.

Selikowitz, S. M., Albala, D. M., Barry, M. J., et al. 1990. Informed patient decision-making: Pilot project (abstract). *Journal of Urology* 4:413A.

Shapiro, S., Venet, W., Strax, P., et al. 1985. Selection, follow-up and analysis in the Health Insurance Plan (HIP) Study. *National Cancer Institute Monographs* 67:65-74.

Tabar, L., Fagerberg, C. J., Gad, A., et al. 1985. Reduction in mortality from breast cancer after mass screening with mammography. *Lancet* 8433:829-832.

Taplin, S. H., Thompson, R. S., Schnitzer, F., et al. 1990. Revisions in the risk-based breast cancer screening program at Group Health Cooperative. *Cancer* 66:812-818.

Thompson, R. S., Carter, A. P., and Taplin, S. H. 1989. Health promotion in an HMO: Ad astra per aspera. *HMO Practice* 3(3):82-88.

Wagner, E. H., and Bledsoe, T. 1990. The Rand health insurance experiment and HMOs. *Medical Care* 28(3):191-200.

Wagner, E. H., and Thompson, R. S. 1988. Cancer prevention and HMOs. *Cancer Investigation* 6:453-459.

Welch, W. P., Hillman, A. L., and Pauly, M. V. 1990. Toward New Typologies for HMOs. *Milbank Memorial Fund Quarterly* 68(2):221-243.

Wilson, J. M. G., and Junger, G. 1968. *Principles and Practice of Screening for Disease.* Public Health Paper No. 34. Geneva, Switzerland: World Health Organization.

5

Cost-Containment Efforts in the Public Sector: Oregon's Priority List

H. Gilbert Welch and Elliott S. Fisher

This paper reviews the most publicized and most controversial portion of Oregon's plan for achieving universal health care coverage—the priority list, released on February 20, 1991, ranking 714 condition-treatment pairs. It discusses the rationale and background for the effort to develop an explicit and comprehensive prioritization of medical services, and it describes the methodology used to develop the list and the public involvement in the process. The paper also offers readers an opportunity to assess the face validity of the final rankings by presenting selected groups of condition-treatment pairs: the extreme high- and low-priority condition-treatment pairs, the priorities assigned to common conditions, the priorities assigned to the different indications for organ transplantation, and a random sampling of condition-treatment pairs. The final portion of the paper briefly discusses both the problems and advantages of public efforts to provide explicit limits on the provision of medical services.

RATIONALE AND BACKGROUND

To ensure that its entire population has health insurance, the Oregon legislature has proposed that all individuals with incomes above the federal poverty level have mandatory workplace coverage and that those with incomes below the poverty level be covered through an expanded Medicaid program. The Medicaid plan uses both of the cost-containment strategies

63

outlined in Chapter 2: global limits and micromanagement. Global limits are imposed by heavy reliance on prepaid capitated care, a strategy that is being increasingly used by other state Medicaid programs (Welch, W. P., 1990). The micromanagement scheme proposed in Oregon, however, is much more controversial and provides the focus for this discussion; it consists of a standard benefit package (for both Medicaid and the mandated workplace coverage) based on an explicit ranking of 714 condition-treatment pairs—better known as Oregon's health care priority list.

The concept of a priority list grew out of a new paradigm of how costs should be contained in state Medicaid programs. The traditional method for dealing with budgetary constraints has been to rely on a combination of strategies: reduced fees to providers, simple limitations in the scope of optional services (such as eliminating dental services), and restrictions in eligibility. It has been assumed, however, that the federally mandated benefit package is fixed. The result has been that the number of covered individuals in most states fluctuates widely, with many individuals losing Medicaid coverage during economic downturns. Oregon proposes that basic Medicaid coverage be guaranteed for the population with incomes below the federal poverty level; that is, the number of beneficiaries should be fixed and benefits should fluctuate instead. Thus, rather than eliminate individuals from the Medicaid rolls in times of budgetary shortfall, Oregon plans to eliminate services from the benefit package. To make such a paradigm operational requires a priority list of medical services.

The process of change was initiated by the 1987 Oregon decision to curtail Medicaid coverage for organ transplantation (Welch, H. G., and Larson, 1988). Funding for bone marrow, heart, liver, and pancreas transplantation was discontinued as part of an effort to provide revenue for an expanded program of basic health care. The trade-off was dramatically framed: the monies required to provide organ transplantation for a projected 34 patients in the biennium would purchase basic health care for 1,500 individuals who had not been covered previously.

But the trade-off was also framed arbitrarily: the state targeted organ transplantation for elimination with little input from the public or from health professionals. Transplantation was chosen because it was an easily identified, new, and expensive therapy that had provided limited benefit (at that time, the 2-year survival rate for state-funded transplant recipients was less than 50 percent) to only a few people. There was little consideration of other health services as a potential source of savings. In 1989, the president of the Oregon state senate responded to these concerns by introducing new legislation. In 1989, Dr. John Kitzhaber authored Senate Bill 27 during the 65th Oregon Legislative Assembly to further expand coverage for basic services and to force a more open, rational, and comprehensive evaluation of the relative value of medical services. The bill established an 11-member Health Services Commission (consisting of five physicians, representing pediatrics, obstetrics, family practice, osteopathic medicine, and public health; four health care consumers; a public health nurse; and a social worker) to oversee implementation of the plan (Welch, H. G., 1989).

RANKING METHODOLOGY

Although Senate Bill 27 specified that public input must be obtained, it left the methodology for establishing priorities to the commission. Public input was sought in three ways.

First, public satisfaction with various health states was obtained from a random telephone survey of Oregonians. Half of the 2,000 individuals contacted were willing to complete the survey. Respondents were asked to rate 6 functional impairments and 23 symptoms. The average weights from the survey are shown in Table 5-1 and are adjusted to a scale of from 0 (death) to 1 (perfect health). The commission speculated that the most surprising result—that loss of consciousness (including fainting, seizures, and coma) was rated as a more satisfactory health state than the taking of prescription medication—was explained by the condition it is most often associated with in an unselected population—a simple faint. Weights for the various health states were used in the net benefit formula described below.

Second, the values ascribed by the public to various treatments (e.g., "treatment of conditions which are fatal and can't be cured—the treatment will not extend the person's life for more than five years," "treatment for alcoholism or drug addiction") were determined during 47 public meetings held across the state. Oregon Health Decisions—a community-based organization that had surveyed the public in the past to identify the relative values placed on health care services (Crawshaw et al., 1990)—organized each meeting. More than a thousand Oregonians attended these meetings; two-thirds were health professionals, and fewer than 50 were Medicaid recipients. The participants were asked to classify each treatment into one of three groups: essential, very important, or important. The fundamental values that guided the foregoing classification were then identified and discussed. The Health Services Commission later combined these values into three general attributes: value to society, value to an individual, and importance to basic health care.

The third approach for soliciting public input, which focused on specific health services, was the sponsorship by the commission of seven public hearings. These hearings allowed special pleading by individuals and advocacy groups and eventually influenced the commission to raise the priority of a few selected services (e.g., preventive dental care).

An initial ranking effort based on a strict, computerized cost-effective-

TABLE 5-1   Weights Assigned to Various Health States Based on
Responses from a Random Telephone Survey of 1,000 Oregonians

Health State	Weight
Functional Impairment	
Unable to drive	.954
In hospital/nursing home	.951
Limited in recreational activity	.938
Need help going to the bathroom or eating	.894
In wheelchair or walker under own control	.627
In bed or wheelchair controlled by someone else	.440
Symptom	
Wear glasses or contact lens	.945
Loss of consciousness (fainting, seizures, coma)	.886
Prescribed medication or diet	.877
Trouble talking	.812
Unable to stop worrying	.785
Overweight or facial acne	.785
Pain in ear/trouble hearing	.783
Trouble falling asleep or staying asleep	.752
Pain or discomfort in eyes	.752
Pain or weakness in back or joints	.747
Difficulty walking	.747
Severe fatigue/weakness	.725
Trouble with sexual performance	.724
Itchy rash over large area	.703
Pain with urination or bowel movement	.701
Headaches or dizziness	.695
Cough/wheezing/trouble breathing	.682
Drainage from sexual organs	.675
Often depressed or upset	.674
Trouble learning or remembering	.633
Stomach ache/vomiting/diarrhea	.630
Severe burn over large area with pain	.628
Trouble with the use of alcohol or drugs	.545

Note: 0 = death; 1 = perfect health. The standard deviation of all weights is < .02.

ness formula produced a preliminary priority list, which was released in
May 1990.   The list ranked 1,600 medical treatments, and it contained
several serious flaws. Effectiveness and cost data were, of course, limited.
But the major problem related more to the cost-effectiveness method itself,
which seemed to favor minor treatments over life-saving ones.   Widely
criticized rankings included the priority of tooth capping over appendecto-
my, reconstructive breast surgery over treatment for open fracture of the
thigh, and treatment for crooked teeth over treatment for Hodgkin's disease.

Transplantation again was near the bottom of the list. Overall, there was widespread unhappiness with the ranking both inside and outside Oregon.

In response, the commission adopted a new approach that modified the foregoing quantitative method by incorporating the consensus views of the commission. The final ranking was the result of three steps. First, to make the ranking more manageable, the commission chose to classify the list of condition-treatment pairs into 17 health service categories, which were then ranked relative to one another. Second, condition-treatment pairs were ranked within each health service category. Third, the 17 separate lists were combined, and those condition-treatment pairs that were judged by the commission to be out of order were reranked.

In step 1, the 17 categories were ranked by summing the weighted category scores derived by each commission member. Before considering individual categories, each commissioner assigned a relative weight (out of a total of 100) to each of the three general attributes identified from the public meetings. The mean weights of the 11 commissioners were as follows: value to society—40 (range: 20 to 60); value to an individual—20 (range: 0 to 40); and importance to basic health care—40 (range: 20 to 50). An individual commissioner's weight was held constant across categories. For each attribute, a commissioner assigned a value of from 1 to 10 to each of the 17 categories. A value of 1 and a value of 10 each had to be assigned to at least one category to ensure a distribution of scores. (A commissioner who had weighted "value to an individual" as only 5, for example, must still have assigned a value of 10 to at least one category for that attribute.) After the initial assignment, category values that were discovered to differ markedly from those of other commissioners could be modified. A summary score for all commissioners was then calculated, which determined the ranking of the 17 categories (Table 5-2).

In step 2, the commissioners worked within categories. They first calculated the net benefit of treatment for each condition-treatment pair. The probability of different outcomes (e.g., death, trouble breathing, need for prescription medicine, return to former health state), both with and without treatment, were incorporated in the net benefit formula:

Net Benefit = [outcomes with treatment × probabilities] –
[outcomes without treatment × probabilities]

Probabilities for death, return to former health state, and intermediate outcomes were multiplied by a value for each health state. The value for death was 0; the value for return to a former health state was 1. Intermediate health states were assigned values obtained from the telephone survey (see Table 5-1).

The ranking of condition-treatment pairs within each category (step 2) was completed by acknowledging the cost of treatment and the number of

TABLE 5-2 Ranking by Members of the Oregon Health Services
Commission of 17 Health Service Categories

Rank   Category Description (number of condition-treatment pairs in category)

1   Acute fatal—treatment prevents death with full recovery (64)
2   Maternity care (53)
3   Acute fatal—treatment prevents death without full recovery (61)
4   Preventive care for children (4)
5   Chronic fatal—treatment improves life span and quality of life (180)
6   Reproductive/contraceptive services (4)
7   Palliative care—death is imminent (2)
8   Preventive dental care (1)
9   Proven effective preventive care for adults (3)
10   Acute nonfatal—treatment allows return to previous health state (60)
11   Chronic nonfatal—one-time treatment improves quality of life (107)
12   Acute nonfatal—treatment without return to previous health state (28)
13   Chronic nonfatal—repetitive treatment improves quality of life (80)
14   Acute nonfatal—treatment expedites recovery from self-limited conditions (31)
15   Infertility services (4)
16   Less effective preventive care for adults (1)
17   Fatal or nonfatal—treatment confers minimal or no improvement in quality of life (31)

individuals who would potentially benefit from the treatment. The commission reordered condition-treatment pairs within a category to account for
these factors. However, they also noted the difficulty of obtaining cost data
in general, the limited ability to determine which costs could reasonably be
attributed to treatment of a condition, and the virtual absence of data on the
costs associated with no treatment. The minimal impact of cost data was
demonstrated by a correlation analysis performed after the final ranking,
which showed no correlation between cost and final rank.

In step 3, the 17 separate priority lists (one for each category) were
entered as blocks into a single document based on their category rank (i.e.,
all condition-treatment pairs in category 1 were placed on top, followed by
those in category 2, etc.). Selected condition-treatment pairs were then reordered "to reflect the clinical and public policy judgement of the Commission" (Oregon Health Services Commission, 1991).

RESULTS

The commission finalized the priority list on February 20, 1991. More
than 60 pages long, it contains 714 condition-treatment pairs. Each entry
includes diagnosis, treatment, the ICD-9 (the World Health Organization's
International Classification of Disease, 9th ed.) code(s) for the listed diag-

TABLE 5-3 Condition-Treatment Pairs with Extreme Rankings

Rank	Category	Condition	Treatment
1	1	Pneumococcal and other bacterial pneumonia	Medical
2	5	Tuberculosis	Medical
3	1	Peritonitis	Medical/surgical
4	1	Foreign body in airways or esophagus	Removal
5	1	Appendicitis	Appendectomy
710	17	Constitutional aplastic anemia[a]	Medical
711	11	Prolapsed urethral mucosa	Surgical
712	17	Central retinal artery occlusion[a]	Paracentesis of aqueous humor
713	17	Extremely low birthweight (< 500 grams) and < 23 weeks' gestation	Life support
714	17	Anencephaly	Life support

[a]Those cases for which treatment confers minimal or no improvement of quality of life.

TABLE 5-4 Ranking for Common Condition-Treatment Pairs

Rank	Category	Condition	Treatment
16	1	Gallstones with cholecystitis	Cholecystectomy
48	3	Acute myocardial infarction	Medical
144	9	Streptococcal sore throat	Medical
176	5	Angina pectoris	Medical/surgical
292	5	Non-life-threatening arrhythmias	Pacemaker
305	5	Chronic obstructive pulmonary disease	Medical
317	11	Hyperplasia of prostate	Transurethral resection
318	5	End-stage renal disease	Dialysis
337	11	Cataract (adult)	Removal
393	11	Osteoarthritis	Arthroplasty
408	11	Transient cerebral ischemia	Endarterectomy
478	13	Osteoarthritis	Medical
502	10	Transient cerebral ischemia	Medical
586	13	Intervertebral disc disorders (back)	Laminectomy
685	17	Gallstones without cholecystitis	Medical/ cholecystectomy
700	14	Acute upper respiratory infections	Medical

nosis, the CPT- 4 (Current Procedural Terminology, 4th ed.) code(s) for the treatment or procedure, the category number, and the rank. The calculated net benefit influenced the final ranking (Pearson correlation coefficient = .47, $p < 0.0001$). The rank of a condition-treatment pair was also strongly

TABLE 5-5 Ranking of the Various Indications for Solid Organ
Transplantation

Rank	Condition	Organ Transplanted
311	End-stage renal disease	Kidney
363	Biliary atresia	Liver
364	Cirrhosis of liver—no mention of alcohol	Liver
365	Myocarditis or pulmonary hypertension	Heart
366	Acute hepatic necrosis	Liver
507	Diabetes and end-stage renal disease	Pancreas/kidney
609	Alpha$_1$-antitrypsin deficiency	Lung
612	Hepatic cancer	Liver
695	Alcoholic liver disease	Liver

Note: All condition-treatment pairs are in category 5, with the exception of acute hepatic
necrosis, which is in category 3.

TABLE 5-6 Ranking of the Various Indications for Bone Marrow
Transplantation and Alternative Therapies

Condition	BMT Rank	Alternative Therapy	Alternative Rank
Hodgkin's disease	208	**Chemotherapy/radiation**	**188**
Acquired aplastic anemia	213	Medical	259
ALL (child)	243	**Chemotherapy/radiation**	**235**
ALL (adult)	243	Chemotherapy/radiation	307
Agranulocytosis	248	None	N.a.
Constitutional aplastic anemia	306	**Medical**	**180**
ANLL	310	Chemotherapy	517
Chronic leukemias	518	**Chemotherapy/radiation**	**278**
Non-Hodgkin's lymphoma	696	**Chemotherapy/radiation**	**238**

Note: Alternative therapies listed in boldface are ranked higher than bone marrow transplantation for the listed indication. All condition-treatment pairs are in category 5.
Abbreviations: BMT, bone marrow transplantation; ALL, acute lymphocytic leukemia; N.a.,
not applicable; ANLL, acute nonlymphocytic leukemia.

influenced by the rank of its health service category (Pearson correlation
coefficient = .83, $p < 0.0001$).

Tables 5-3 through 5-7 give the reader a feeling for the final ranking as
well as an opportunity to consider its face validity. Table 5-3 shows the
condition-treatment pairs ranked at both extremes (the five highest and the
five lowest ranks). Antibiotic therapy for bacterial pneumonia tops the list;

TABLE 5-7 Ten Randomly Selected Condition-Treatment Pairs

Rank	Category	Condition	Treatment
86	3	Subarachnoid and intercerebral hemorrhage	Burr holes/ craniotomy
246	5	Pernicious anemia	Medical
254	5	Opportunistic infections in immunocompromised hosts	Medical
273	5	Regional enteritis	Medical/surgical
383	13	Cerebral palsy	Medical
490	11	Ganglion of tendon or joint	Excision
494	5	Histiocytosis	Medical
520	5	Anomalies of the gallbladder, bile ducts, and liver	Medical/surgical
674	14	Acute pharyngitis and laryngitis	Medical
706	17	Cyst of the kidney (acquired)	Medical/surgical

life support for a newborn with anencephaly is at the bottom. Table 5-4 shows the rankings for common condition-treatment pairs. For the two conditions for which medical and surgical treatment are listed separately, surgical therapy has the higher rank. Arthroplasty (e.g., hip replacement) has higher priority than medical therapy for osteoarthritis; endarterectomy has higher priority than medical therapy for cerebral ischemia.

The motivation for the priority list was, in part, the recognition that the decision to curtail funding for organ transplantation had been arbitrary. Tables 5-5 and 5-6 demonstrate that organ transplantation is no longer at the bottom of the list. Table 5-5 shows the rankings of various indications for solid organ transplantation. These ranks were, in general, lower than those for bone marrow transplantation. Table 5-6 demonstrates the level of detail used by the Health Services Commission for this single procedure. Nine indications for marrow transplantation are shown, as are eight alternative treatment strategies. Five of the alternative treatments (boldface) have a higher rank than marrow transplantation.

Finally, to offer the reader an unselected sample, Table 5-7 includes 10 condition-treatment pairs drawn at random.

DISCUSSION

The level of funding provided by the Oregon state legislature will ultimately determine which condition-treatment pairs are covered. The resulting benefit package, once a federal waiver is approved, will apply to the Medicaid program and will also serve as the minimum benefit package to be offered under the mandated employer-based insurance. Despite the fact that the results of the priority list may only apply to a segment of the population, the Oregon experience deserves scrutiny for its potential relevance to a more universal health insurance plan.

The mandate of the Oregon Legislative Assembly to develop a "list of health services ranked from the most important to the least important" is a particularly daunting task. Because no prototype was available for guidance, the Health Services Commission was forced to break new ground. Thousands of volunteer hours were devoted to the process by both professionals and ordinary citizens. The community meetings and telephone surveys represent a level of public input rarely solicited in health policy planning. Any health professional who reviews this process will be impressed by the effort committed to the task.

But they will be equally impressed by the problems facing this kind of micromanagement. Three are particularly noteworthy. The first is accuracy. Adapting either cost-effectiveness analysis or a consensus approach to such a comprehensive task was bound to be fraught with problems. For many condition-treatment pairs there are few data on effectiveness, a problem compounded by the difficulty of comparing dissimilar benefits. Whereas the extreme high and low ranks shown in Table 5-3 have legitimate face validity, the relative priorities of more closely ranked services are, with good reason, open to question. For example, the higher priority (rank = 318) assigned to treatment for end-stage renal disease in comparison with treatment for cataracts (rank = 337; see Table 5-4) may engender vigorous debate. Furthermore, because a line must ultimately be drawn, the accuracy of adjacent ranks is relative. For example, in Table 5-5, is it appropriate to fund heart transplantation for myocarditis (rank = 365) and not fund liver transplantation for acute hepatic necrosis (rank = 366)? Because the available data were limited and the methodologies not sufficiently mature, the commission was forced to make decisions that in retrospect appear arbitrary and may not be reproducible.

More important is the problem of heterogeneity. Even if perfect data were available and a consensus about the rankings could be obtained, exceptions would exist. Priorities that make sense for the population as a whole may fail miserably for the specific case. Although internists may be unhappy to learn that arthroplasty (rank = 393) is more valued than ibuprofen (rank = 478) in the treatment of osteoarthritis, it may be defensible to rank definitive treatment over palliation. For a patient with mild pain or one with extreme surgical risk, however, it is farcical. In addition, the heterogeneity of patient preferences is relevant (Barry et al., 1988). The ranking of surgical procedures above their medical alternatives ignores those patients who may prefer less invasive therapy. Although it is easy for clinicians to imagine such exceptions, it is difficult for policymakers to incorporate them into a set of priorities.

Finally, there is the problem of administration. Since the priorities are catalogued by diagnosis, physician discretion in the choice of diagnosis could have a dramatic impact on the rank assigned their therapy. Some consideration must be given to the problem of "gaming" by physicians, particularly if financial incentives to do so persist. Will cultures be required to ensure that physicians are treating strep pharyngitis (rank = 144) and not the common cold (rank = 700)? How can cholecystectomies for symptomatic cholelithiasis (rank = 16) be distinguished from those for asymptomatic stones (rank = 685)? The incentives for providers to inflate diagnoses will be powerful when rank determines whether reimbursement occurs. Furthermore, it is unclear how a priority list can deal with patients whose symptoms have yet to be diagnosed or whose diagnosis does not appear on the list.

Recognition of these problems has led Oregon's legislative leaders to emphasize a strategy that combines the priority list with capitation. In essence, however, it is a strategy that combines micromanagement with global limits. The priority list will define the benefit package on which the capitated rate will be based. Physicians will be free to prescribe treatments outside the benefit package but with no increase in total reimbursement. This approach will go a long way toward solving the problem of heterogeneity—by allowing for a more flexible allocation process tailored to the individual patient. By addressing incentives directly, capitation should lessen the problem of gaming. How capitated health systems will actually implement the priority list, however, remains unknown. Where capitation is impractical (e.g., rural Oregon), the problems of heterogeneity and administration are likely to be more severe. Clearly, regardless of reimbursement strategy, implementation of a priority list in clinical practice will be difficult.

On the other hand, there are certain aspects of a priority list that would offer benefits to physicians. The current pressures for cost containment force the health care system and the nation to face the problem of which services to deliver and to whom. Societal guidance about these choices would be appreciated, for two major reasons. The first is to mitigate the problem of malpractice by establishing agreed-upon standards of care that recognize the current environment of limited resources. Second, and more importantly, a system of public priorities will provide the ethical foundation needed to curtail services with token or undetermined benefit. A public policy not to support extremely low birthweight infants (rank = 713) could serve as an important example.

In addition, a priority list might benefit society as well. Such a list forces explicit decisions about how to use limited resources and encourages public scrutiny of the process employed to make those decisions. Currently, much of this decision making is underground, and resource allocation decisions vary considerably. Because decisions are neither standardized nor publicized, there is little opportunity for public input. Application of a priority list within a universal health insurance plan might mitigate such problems.

The need to set limits in health care coverage is sufficiently acute to warrant a consideration of priority setting, despite its problems. Admittedly, many refinements are needed. A more comprehensive approach will require evaluation of more condition-treatment pairs. The RAND Corporation, for example, defined 864 distinct indications for carotid endarterectomy alone (Chassin et al., 1987). The problem of whose set of utilities are used to define health states also needs attention. The tension between using an unselected population (which may have minimal symptom experience) and diseased populations (which may have a tendency to inflate those symptoms they would experience without treatment) will have to be addressed (Mulley, 1989). More consideration should also be given to the measurement of cost. Eventually, incremental cost must be calculated with careful consideration given to what is chosen as alternative therapy (Detsky and Naglie, 1990). And, of course, more and better data are needed.

Finally, given the objectives of this volume, the relationship between priority setting and technological innovation requires exploration. It is possible that the process of establishing priorities may change the rate of technological advance; it is also possible that technological advances will drive new priorities. The latter is certainly the case for a single state, whose health policy can have only minimal impact on innovation in medicine. On the one hand, Oregon has acknowledged the potential impact of new technologies on the priorities it has already established and intends periodically to reconsider its rankings. On the other hand, a widely applied priority list could influence the rate of technological advance—with research on low-priority conditions and treatments deemphasized. Although the rate of technological innovation is largely determined by the resources that are available, explicit priorities may govern where innovation occurs.

Explicit priority setting has an important contribution to make in determining what health care services to purchase in an era of limited budgets. It is especially relevant to health systems working within global limits, such as Britain's National Health Service (see Chapter 6). The efforts being made in Oregon ought to advance this process. The state's approach has and will continue to foster vigorous debate (Duggan, 1989; Gore, 1990; Relman, 1990; Schwartz and Aaron, 1990; Hollingsbaum, 1991). The methodology used to create the priority list is likely to undergo extensive peer review. The ranks of individual condition-treatment pairs undoubtedly will be a source of considerable dispute, encouraging further efficacy and cost-effectiveness research. Finally, Oregon's efforts should encourage those who say such a method is unworkable to develop some alternative.

ACKNOWLEDGMENTS

The authors appreciate the efforts of W. Pete Welch, Ph.D., and Jennifer Dixon, M.D., for their assistance in this work. In addition, they are particularly indebted to the staff of the Oregon Health Services Commission and the Oregon Senate President's Office who were exceptionally responsive to requests for information.

REFERENCES

Barry, M. J., Mulley, A. G. Jr., Fowler, F. J., and Wennberg, J. E. 1988. Watchful waiting vs. immediate transurethral resection for symptomatic prostatism: The importance of patients' preferences. *Journal of the American Medical Association* 259:3010-3017.

Chassin, M. R., Kosecoff, J., Park, R. E., et al. 1987. Does inappropriate use explain geographic variations in the use of health care services? A study of three procedures. *Journal of the American Medical Association* 258:2533-2537.

Crawshaw, R., Garland, M., Hines, B., and Anderson, D. 1990. Developing principles for prudent health care allocation: The continuing Oregon experiment. *Western Journal of Medicine* 321:1261-1264.

Detsky, A. S., and Naglie, I. G. 1990. A clinician's guide to cost-effectiveness analysis. *Annals of Internal Medicine* 113:147-154.

Duggan, J. M. 1989. Resource allocation and bioethics. *Lancet* 1:772-773.

Gore, A. 1990. Oregon's bold mistake. *Academic Medicine* 65:634-635.

Hollingsbaum, F. 1991. Rationing health care. *British Medical Journal* 302:288-289.

Mulley, A. G. Jr. 1989. Assessing patients' utilities: Can the ends justify the means? *Medical Care* 27:S269-S281.

Oregon Health Services Commission. 1991. Prioritized Health Services List of February 20, 1991. Salem, Ore.: The Commission.

Relman, A. 1990. The trouble with rationing. *New England Journal of Medicine* 323:911-912.

Schwartz, W., and Aaron, H. 1990. The Achilles heel of health care rationing. *New York Times*, July 9.

Welch, H. G. 1989. Health care tickets for the uninsured—first class, coach, or standby? *New England Journal of Medicine* 321:1261-1264.

Welch, H. G., and Larson, E. B. 1988. Dealing with limited resources: The Oregon decision to curtail funding for organ transplantation. *New England Journal of Medicine* 319:171-173.

Welch, W. P. 1990. Giving physicians incentives to contain costs under Medicaid. *Health Care Financing Review* 12(Winter):103-112.

Part III
Managing Care in the United Kingdom and Canada

6

Priority Setting in a
Needs-based System

Alan Williams

The British health care system is of particular interest because it has, from its inception in 1948, sought to reconcile widespread access to health care with a tight, centrally controlled budget. Before considering how well or ill it has performed in that respect, certain key features need to be borne in mind:

1. The National Health Service (NHS) is committed to providing care according to need, not according to willingness or ability to pay. It works within a strong, but ill-defined, egalitarian ideology.

2. The NHS provides about 90 percent of all health care for British citizens; the private sector concentrates mainly on providing elective surgery for those who wish to avoid NHS waiting lists and for those who wish to improve on the general level of hospital amenities. Private treatment is provided in large part by doctors who spend most of their time in the NHS.

3. The NHS has a centrally determined, tax-financed, fixed annual budget, which is distributed geographically to regional (and district) health authorities. Distribution follows a formula based mostly on (weighted) population but to some extent also on geographic variations in deprivation and morbidity/mortality rates. These health authorities are responsible for the provision of all the health care in their area and for coordinating the provision of domiciliary support services with local authorities (see below).

4. The total NHS budget is approximately 6 percent of the gross national product (GNP), of which approximately 60 percent is spent on hospital services. Local authorities, who are formally outside this centrally tax-financed system, provide many health-related services for the domiciliary support of ill and disabled people (services that are very important in the care of the elderly and certain other vulnerable groups).

5. Apart from accidents and emergencies, the patient's first point of contact is always with the general practitioner (GP), who acts as the "gatekeeper" for the system. Every patient is registered with a GP (in principle if not in practice). Under the NHS system, there are small charges for primary care prescriptions, somewhat larger charges for dental and ophthalmic services, and no charges for hospital care. Thus, billing is totally absent, which significantly reduces both the system's administrative overhead and its knowledge of how much things cost. NHS hospital doctors are salaried employees, and GPs are independent contractors, most of whose salaries come from capitation fees paid for the patients registered with them. Fee-for-service charges are rare; they are used only when it is desirable to encourage specific activities (such as home visits or night calls).

6. Political support for this system is strong among the public and among health care providers. The system, however, is widely believed to be underfunded and forced to make painful decisions that it is thought could be avoided if funding could be increased.

PROBLEMS OF THE BRITISH HEALTH CARE SYSTEM

It will be obvious from the above that the British health care system has no problem with cost containment, if by that is meant controlling *total* costs. Instead, two other issues predominate: (1) is the right amount being spent on health care? and (2) is good value being received for the money that is spent? The present state of knowledge about the marginal benefits of health care spending precludes an accurate answer to the first question. The second question is more interesting, and most of this paper will be devoted to addressing it and exploring its ramifications. The broad response of most observers to this question is that surprisingly good results are achieved, considering how little is put into the system. Others might argue, this author among them, that the results are good largely *because* so little is put in.

Before considering the way the system works, some general observations are in order about optimization subject to constraints (i.e., about the discipline of economics). The resources devoted to health care must be diverted from other valuable uses; therefore, it is not rational to extend health care provision to the point where *all* the good that could be done is being done. The system should stop providing health care when the extra health benefit to be gained is of approximately the same value as whatever has been given up to provide the extra resources for health care. This principle demands that health care alternatives be ranked in order of cost-effectiveness; in a system with a fixed budget, the choosing of which services to fund proceeds by starting at the top of the list and working down it until the point in this priority ordering at which the money runs out. Once the system's budget level is set, the optimization problem is one of establishing (and implementing) priorities in cost-effectiveness terms.

It is here that this paper's first background point becomes crucial. In a private health care system that seeks profitability (or at least to break even), optimization requires that alternatives be subjected to *financial* appraisal—that is, to systematic analysis of the revenue and expenditure implications of each alternative. The precise pattern of the rationing that ensues will be the result of (somebody's) willingness and ability to meet (at least) the estimated expenditures. Here, the "somebody" may be an individual, an insurer, a charity or foundation, or a public agency, and they may or may not be in a position to judge the likely effectiveness of treatment when deciding how much to pay. In fact, the multiplicity of actors in this system is likely to lead to great variability in such judgments. But in a public system that has explicitly rejected willingness and ability to pay as a rationing device, and that has its revenue fixed according to the population for which it is responsible (rather than according to what it does for them), optimization needs to be informed by *economic* appraisal. That is, it should be guided by systematic analysis of the benefit and cost implications of alternatives; rationing thus will be guided by (somebody's) assessment of a person's ability to benefit (i.e., by "need" for treatment) in relation to the costs (which will be borne by the citizenry at large). In practice, these economic appraisals have unfortunately limited their consideration of cost implications to the implications for the NHS budget (because that is the constraint uppermost in people's minds), and in practice, the "somebody" who assesses need, at both the clinical and community levels, has for the most part been a doctor. To do this job properly, doctors should know not only about the effectiveness (in outcome terms) of the treatments at their disposal, and how their patients value these various outcomes, but also about the benefits of all the other treatments the system provides for other patients, and how benefits to one patient are to be weighed against benefits to another. Needless to say, no one has this information, but doctors believe that because of their clinical experience they are best placed to fill the void. Consequently, it has been their priorities that have driven the system (with little regard to costs). Concern about costs has been left to the managers in the health authorities or in the hospitals, who, because they had little or no influence over (or even knowledge about) the priorities that were being applied by doctors in the use of the system's capacity, found themselves having to make rather arbitrary decisions about increasing or decreasing that capacity, in order to balance their predetermined (fixed) budgets.

The gatekeeper role mentioned in point number 5 at the beginning of this chapter requires the GP to be the initial "needs-assessor" (once the patient has decided that he or she "needs" to see a doctor, i.e., that he or she might benefit from such an encounter). If the GP refers the patient to a hospital doctor, a second needs assessment takes place, and at this point an important conflict of interest manifests itself. Can the doctor simultaneously act as the patient's agent and the system's agent? Or, to put the point differently, should the doctor be expected to mediate the conflict between the interests of the citizen-as-taxpayer (in keeping costs down) and the interests of the citizen-as-patient (in getting the best possible "free" care)? Can he or she do so evenhandedly, when the citizen-as-patient is sitting there and the citizen-as-taxpayer is vicariously represented only by a busy, somewhat remote manager who is rather detached from the pressures of clinical work and probably located in a different building? Although the majority of British doctors seem comfortable with this role most of the time, every now and again a protest is heard; occasionally, a doctor asserts that it is his role to do everything he can for the patient in front of him, no matter what the cost, and that that is what he proposes to do, because for him to do anything else would be unethical.

A brief excursion into medical ethics seems called for here. Put succinctly, medical ethics require a doctor to do no harm, to preserve life, to alleviate suffering, to respect the autonomy of the patient, to tell the truth, and to deal fairly with patients. It is accepted that these principles often conflict and that one of the skills required of doctors is to exercise appropriate judgment as to where to strike a compromise between them in any particular clinical situation. The injunction to deal fairly with patients differs from the others in that it requires a comparison to be made between what is done for one person and what is done for another. In a regime of fixed budgets, to offer a treatment to one person, *regardless of the cost of that treatment*, implies that no account is to be paid to the inescapable consequence that some other patients will be denied treatment, and that those sacrifices by others will be commensurate with the costs that are being disregarded. This approach is not consistent with "dealing fairly" with patients, which, at the very least, requires that the needs of other potential patients be weighed in the balance of treatment decisions. Thus, the argument that it is unethical for doctors to play the gatekeeper role is untenable (which is not to deny that the role might actually be played in an unethical way by some doctors).

Let us return to the main theme, however, which is the setting of priorities in a needs-driven system. As will be evident from the foregoing, *need* is defined as the capacity to benefit (people cannot need something that is of no benefit to them). But the capacity to benefit from any health care activity varies (among treatments, among patients, and even among practitioners) and might be so small in relation to its costs as not to be worth providing. In other words, needs must be prioritized, and some will, inevitably and quite properly, remain unmet. Thus, if the people on waiting lists are those whose capacity to benefit from treatment is smaller than those who are not kept waiting, this constitutes evidence that the system is working rationally (not that it has failed nor that it needs more money, for even with more money there would still be marginal cases on waiting lists). A more legitimate cause for concern would arise if those on waiting lists would benefit more from early treatment than many of the people who were not being forced to wait. The general point remains, however: the mere existence of waiting lists, or their size, or even the length of the wait, is not important. What is important is the size of the benefits that are being denied to those who are waiting, compared with what other people are receiving—that is, a comparison of needs.

It is necessary to determine how benefits are to be measured in a need-driven system. The first factor to keep in mind is that what people want is not treatment per se but improved health. Improved health means the extension of one's life expectancy or a better quality of life, or both. Because each is valued, people may be willing to trade off one against the other. Health-related quality of life is judged by examining such characteristics as mobility, self-care, pain, distress, and ability to perform normal, accustomed social (including work) roles. Measuring the benefits of treatment requires estimates of the effect of treatment on these various characteristics of health, which, in principle, are encapsulated in the concept of the quality-adjusted life year (or QALY). Yet disappointingly little is known in these terms about the health benefits to be derived from most treatment for most people. So at the very heart of the priority-setting process is a great information void, which renders the system vulnerable to priority setting by less appropriate means. The recent discovery and promotion of outcomes research is a belated response to this information void.

THE "REFORMED" BRITISH HEALTH CARE SYSTEM

On All Fools Day 1991, the reforms of the NHS that had been instituted by the Thatcher government went into effect. Their principal feature is the separation of the demand side of the market for health care from the supply side. On the supply side (the providers) are the hospitals, the primary care doctors, and the community services. On the demand side (the purchasers) are the health authorities and those GPs who have been permitted to become budget-holders.[1] There are some obvious anomalies here, such as the am-

---

[1]This means that certain large group practices will receive part of the hospital budget, which allows their GPs to purchase certain hospital services on behalf of their patients.

biguous role of primary care doctors and the designation of community services as providers when they are not really part of the system at all but are run by local authorities. (Despite recommendations that the government received to expand and strengthen the community care system, Mrs. Thatcher prevaricated in regard to this because she could not agree to any strengthening of the role of local government in Britain.) There are also some less obvious anomalies—for example, certain hospitals (and a few other providers) enjoy a special status as self-governing trusts, which exempts them from some of the restrictions (e.g., on pay and conditions of staff, access to capital, etc.) placed on hospitals that remain within the main NHS system. Generally, however, the idea is that providers will compete with each other for contracts drawn up by the purchasers, who will choose the provider that offers the best deal.

Each purchaser's task is to assess the need of the particular population for which it is responsible, set performance criteria for potential providers (which should relate to quality as well as quantity), and evaluate the bids against policy objectives and budget constraints. Certain services (e.g., accident and emergency) must be provided locally, but others (especially elective surgery) might be "bought in" from hospitals outside the geographic boundaries of the purchasing health authority.

Clearly, this kind of competition is more viable in large urban areas than in more sparsely populated areas, and it depends on the providers' not forming informal cartels. More crucially, however, it depends on the ability of purchasers to specify the content of contracts in the manner required, which leads one to the information void mentioned earlier. If need means capacity to benefit, purchasers must know what is beneficial and what is not, and just how beneficial the beneficial things are in relation to the costs. They must also monitor performance in outcome (rather than process) terms, a task of no small difficulty, given a situation in which even medical audits directed at technical competence have been voluntary, nonthreatening educational activities pursued only by enthusiasts who set their own local standards and operate in a rather informal (and highly secretive) manner. Even now the official position is that audits are to be strictly professional affairs in which managers are not to be told anything that might enable them to identify individuals who are performing poorly. It is likely to take at least a decade to generate a data base that will enable any of these changes to operate in a manner that is even passably systematic, and for the first few years, even with determination and goodwill, the reforms are unlikely to move beyond the level of ritual.

In the new system, the rationing or priority-setting role is vested firmly in the purchasers, but to make their chosen priorities effective they will have to specify the case-mix of each hospital specialty and check on patient selection criteria and quality of performance. It is not clear quite how this is going to happen if the rhetoric surrounding the protection of clinical freedom and the voluntary and confidential nature of medical audits is to be taken seriously. Making doctors budget-holders may force them to think in terms of priorities and cost-effectiveness, but it will not necessarily lead them to adopt the particular priorities, or notions of effectiveness, held by the health authorities.

IMPLICATIONS FOR TECHNOLOGICAL ADVANCE IN MEDICINE

In principle, it is clear that what makes a technological innovation a technological advance is that it proves to be beneficial in cost-per-QALY terms. To determine whether an innovation can make such a leap in status, it should be introduced initially in a controlled manner in which it is used only in the context of a carefully designed evaluative trial that is conducted by independent researchers, with full disclosure of data, and financed outside the main therapeutic budget of the health service. Only when such a test has been passed should the innovation move into the armamentarium of practicing clinicians, and possibly even then only with restrictions on its use.

But it is necessary here to distinguish between those innovations that require the use of (expensive) specialized resources, be they drugs, devices, or people, and those that can easily be accommodated within the existing resources for everyday clinical activities. In the latter case, there are few effective sanctions that can be applied at a managerial level to enforce independent evaluation, and the only early indicator that something different is happening may be a change in patient selection, as an interested clinician seeks more cases on whom to practice the innovation. In the British system, this is most likely to be noticed if the waiting lists for certain conditions lengthen because these cases have been squeezed out to make room for the innovative ones. Health authorities have learned, when new appointments are made, to monitor as closely as possible the likely implications of clinicians' research interests.

Even if formal evaluation could be enforced prior to general dissemination of an innovative practice, there are some obvious disadvantages, mainly to do with delay. It may take quite a while to establish rigorously a clear gain to patients, and even longer to be sure that there are no adverse effects over the longer term. Given the variety and complexity of manufacturers' pricing policies, it may not be easy to extrapolate from the cost data in the trial to the costs that are likely to be faced when the innovation becomes more widely disseminated. Indeed, if it is known that a particular cost-effectiveness ratio has been established by purchasers as the cutoff point between what can be afforded and what cannot, manufacturers may well use the results of the trial to price the technology at a level that is as close to that ratio as possible, even though the true cost of producing it is much lower. An additional problem common to all trials is that the results obtained by well-disciplined practitioners observing punctiliously the protocol of a scientific trial may not be replicated when the technology is being used in the "real world" of clinical practice. Nevertheless, the system does have to move in the direction of earlier, more formal cost-effectiveness analysis of emerging new technologies. One sign that this has already been accepted is the current burgeoning interest of the drug companies in quality of life measurement and cost-effectiveness analysis. Inevitably, however, their interest is more strongly motivated by marketing considerations than by a desire to improve the efficiency of the health care system or to enhance the methodology of cost-effectiveness analysis, although both of those beneficial side effects may follow incidentally.

The increasing pressure for earlier and more formal economic appraisal has come from dissatisfaction with the existing situation. Health authorities see themselves confronting collusive activity among manufacturers, practitioners, and patients, which prevents or delays systematic evaluation and leads to the weakly controlled dissemination of well-marketed but poorly evaluated new technologies. Manufacturers encourage and exploit the desire of practitioners to improve their performance by offering something that helps them resolve some diagnostic, monitoring, or therapeutic difficulty of which they are acutely aware, given the current state of the art of medical practice in their particular field. In addition to the desire to help their patients, practitioners are motivated to pursue innovative technologies by the various professional "perks" associated with them, such as subsidized attendance at professional conferences in sometimes delightful locations and personal association with published research findings. The patients themselves can usually be induced to go along with the latest "advance" (especially if it has also been promoted in the media as the latest technological wonder). NHS qualms about the costs of, say, radiological equipment (which nowadays may include qualms about the associated operating expenses as well as about capital costs) can be overcome by "giving" the capacity to the service during the experimental phase. Unless it proves to be positively harmful, the technology becomes incorporated into routine practice in the experimental sites, and possibly elsewhere, through the influential grapevine of the conference circuit. By the time the stage is reached when the health authority itself has to pick up the costs, it will have become politically quite difficult to discontinue it on cost-effectiveness grounds, especially if the media can show a handful of people who have benefited dramatically from the innovation. The constraint of its fixed budget has made the British system notoriously slow, compared with most countries of equivalent wealth, in diffusing expensive new technologies throughout the system. Yet that very system also offers opportunities, by virtue of its monopsonistic position within the United Kingdom, for guiding this diffusion in a purposeful way. Unfortunately, effective strategies by which to exploit these opportunities have yet to be developed.

RATIONING HEALTH CARE: IS IT ETHICAL?

This much-asked question is always puzzling because it is so oddly formulated. If by *rationing* is meant deciding who is to get something and who is to go without, then rationing, like death, is unavoidable. No one asks, is death ethical? Instead, practitioners do (and should) ask, when they have some influence over the situation, whether it is ethical to allow (or cause) someone to die in a particular manner at a particular time rather than in some other manner at some other time. So it should be with rationing. The appropriate question is whether it is ethical to impose a particular kind of rationing on a particular community at a particular time, as opposed to imposing some other kind of rationing on that community at that time.

Before answering this question, it is necessary to examine the particular ideology that a community wishes to bring to bear on its health care system. Essentially two such ideologies are relevant in this context, the libertarian and the egalitarian. In the libertarian view, access to health care is part of the society's reward system, and as a general rule, people should be able to use their income and wealth to get more or better health care than their fellow citizens, should they so wish. In the egalitarian view, access to health care is every citizen's right (like access to the ballot box or to the courts of justice), and it ought not to be influenced by income or wealth. Each of these broad viewpoints is typically associated with a distinctive configuration of views on personal responsibility, social concern, freedom, and equality, as set out in Table 6-1.

The ascendancy of either of these broad viewpoints would generate a distinctive health care system whose characteristics would be very different from those of a system shaped by the other viewpoint. A system shaped by the libertarian ideology would establish willingness and ability to pay as the determinants of access; this kind of access would be best accomplished through a market-oriented "private" system (provided such markets can be kept competitive). In an egalitarian system, equal opportunity of access for those in equal need would be the determining rule, and because this requires the establishment of a social hierarchy of need independent of who is paying for the care, it would be best implemented through a system of public provision of care (provided the system can be kept responsive to social values and changing economic circumstances). Table 6-2 lists the essential characteristics of each kind of idealized system. Note that the success criterion to be applied to the egalitarian system is the level and distribution of *health* in the community.

TABLE 6-1   Attitudes Typically Associated with the Libertarian and
Egalitarian Viewpoints

Issue	Libertarian Viewpoint	Egalitarian Viewpoint
Personal responsibility	Personal responsibility for achievement is very important, and this quality is weakened if people are offered unearned rewards. Moreover, such unearned rewards weaken the motivational force that ensures economic well-being; in so doing, they also undermine moral well-being, because of the intimate connection between moral well-being and personal efforts to achieve.	Personal incentives to achieve are desirable, but economic failure is not equated with moral depravity or social worthlessness.
Social concern	Social Darwinism dictates a seemingly cruel indifference to the fate of those who cannot "make the grade." A less extreme position is that charity, expressed and effected preferably under private auspices, is the proper vehicle; however, charity should be exercised under carefully prescribed conditions, for example, such that the potential recipient must first mobilize his or her own resources and, when helped, must not be in as favorable a position as those who are self-supporting (the principle of "lesser eligibility").	Private charitable action is not rejected but is seen as potentially dangerous morally (because it is often demeaning to the recipient and corrupting to the donor) and usually inequitable. It seems preferable to establish social mechanisms that create and sustain self-sufficiency and that are accessible according to precise rules concerning entitlement, which are applied equitably and are explicitly sanctioned by society at large.
Freedom	Freedom is to be sought as a supreme good in itself. Compulsion attenuates both personal responsibility and individualistic and voluntary expressions of social concern. Centralized health	Freedom is seen as the presence of real opportunities of choice; although economic constraints are less openly coercive than political constraints, they are nonetheless real and often constitute the effective limits on choice.

continued

TABLE 6-1 *Continued*

Issue	Libertarian Viewpoint	Egalitarian Viewpoint
	planning and a large governmental role in health care financing are seen as an unwarranted abridgment of the freedom of patients as well as of health professionals, and private medicine is thereby viewed as a bulwark against totalitarianism.	Freedom is not indivisible but may be sacrificed in one respect to obtain greater freedom in some other. Government is not an external threat to individuals in the society but is the means by which individuals achieve greater scope for action (that is, greater real freedom).
Equality	Equality before the law is the key concept, with clear precedence being given to freedom over equality whenever the two conflict.	The only moral justification for using personal achievement as the basis for distributing rewards is the availability of equal opportunities for such achievement for all individuals. Emphasis is then placed on equality of opportunity; where this cannot be ensured, the moral worth of achievement is undermined. Equality is seen as an extension to the many of the freedom actually enjoyed by only the few.

SOURCE: Based on A. Williams, "Priority Setting in Public and Private Health Care: A Guide Through the Ideological Jungle," *Journal of Health Economics* 7:173-183, 1988.

Needless to say, in practice neither system fully lives up to its ideals. Most of the problems stem from (1) the peculiar role of doctors in health care systems, (2) market deficiencies on the supply side, and (3) difficulties with information on the demand side. Table 6-3 catalogues the full extent of these problems.

In most countries health care is provided through a mixture of systems that have no common ideology, which is probably a reflection of the pluralized societies of those nations and their attempts to accommodate subgroups with incompatible systems of beliefs. A hypothesis suggested by this analysis is that the structure of the health care system in each country is likely to be systematically related to the equity concerns that have been dominant in the recent past; the health care system is also likely to reflect the ideology that generated those concerns. An obvious instance is the balance be-

TABLE 6-2   Essential Characteristics of Idealized Health Care Systems
Based on Libertarian Views (Private Systems) and Egalitarian Views
(Public Systems)

System Element	Private Systems	Public Systems
Demand	• Individuals are the best judges of their own welfare.	• When ill, individuals are frequently imperfect judges of their own welfare.
	• Priorities are determined by people's own willingness and ability to pay.	• Priorities are determined by social judgments about need.
	• The erratic and potentially catastrophic nature of demand is mediated by private insurance.	• The erratic and potentially catastrophic nature of demand is made irrelevant by the provision of free services.
	• Matters of equity are dealt with elsewhere (e.g., in the tax and social security systems).	• Since the distribution of income and wealth is unlikely to be equitable in relation to the need for health care, the system must be insulated from its influence.
Supply	• Profit is the proper and most effective way to motivate suppliers to respond to the needs of demanders.	• Professional ethics and dedication to public service are the appropriate motivation of suppliers, who should focus on success in curing or caring.
	• Priorities are determined by people's willingness and ability to pay and by the costs of meeting their wishes at the margin.	• Priorities are determined by identifying the greatest improvements in caring or curing that can be effected at the margin.
	• Suppliers have a strong incentive to adopt least-cost methods of service provision.	• Predetermined limits on available resources create a strong incentive for suppliers to adopt least-cost methods of service provision.
Adjustment mechanism(s)	• Many competing suppliers ensure that prices are kept low and reflect costs.	• Central review of activities generates efficiency audits of service provision; management pressures keep the system cost-effective.
	• Well-informed consumers are able to seek out the most	• Well-informed clinicians are able to prescribe the most

continued

TABLE 6-2 *Continued*

System Element	Private Systems	Public Systems
	cost-effective form of treatment for themselves. • If medical practice is profitable at the price that prevails in the market, more people will go into medicine; hence, supply will be demand responsive. If, conversely, medical practice is unremunerative, people will leave it, or stop entering it, until the system returns to equilibrium.	cost-effective form of treatment for each patient. • If there is demand pressure on some facilities or specialties, resources will be directed toward extending them. Facilities or specialties on which demand pressure is slack will be slimmed down to release resources for other uses.
Success criteria	• Consumers will judge the system by their ability to get someone to do what they demand, when, where, and how they want it done. • Producers will judge the system by how substantial a living they can make through it.	• The electorate judges the system by the extent to which it improves the health status of the population at large in relation to the resources allocated to it. • Producers judge the system by its ability to enable them to provide the treatments they believe to be cost-effective.

SOURCE: Based on A. Williams, "Priority Setting in Public and Private Health Care: A Guide Through the Ideological Jungle," *Journal of Health Economics* 7:173-183, 1988.

tween public and private provision of care, which differs markedly among countries.

It was recently observed that Americans regard the British system (of rationing) as unacceptably coercive because it prevents people from getting the care they want and are willing to pay for; the British, on the other hand, consider the American system (of rationing) unacceptably coercive because it denies some people access to services that are available to others with similar needs. Perhaps the answer to the ethical question should be that each system is better than the other if one applies that system's own avowed criterion. Those seeking reform of either system may be reflecting one of the following viewpoints: (1) they want their system to reflect a different ideological position from the one on which it is currently based, and from that new position their own system appears deficient and should therefore be changed; or (2) their system does not perform very well according to its own ideological tenets and should be reformed to embody its ideals more

TABLE 6-3   Characteristics of Actual Private and Public Health Care
Systems

System Element	Private Systems	Public Systems
Demand	• Doctors act as agents, mediating demand on behalf of consumers. • Priorities are determined by the reimbursement rules of insurance funds.	• Doctors act as agents, identifying need on behalf of patients. • Priorities are determined by the doctor's own professional situation, by his or her assessment of the patient's condition, and by the expected trouble-making proclivities of the patient.
	• Because private insurance coverage is itself a profit-seeking activity, some risk rating is inevitable; consequently, coverage is incomplete and uneven, distorting personal willingness and ability to pay. • Attempts to change the distribution of income and wealth independently are resisted as destroying incentives (one of which is the ability of the rich to buy better or more medical care).	• Freedom from direct financial contributions at the point of service and the absence of risk rating enable patients to seek treatment for trivial or inappropriate conditions. • Attempts to correct inequities in the social and economic system by differential compensatory access to health services lead to recourse to health care in circumstances in which it is unlikely to be a cost-effective solution to the problem.
Supply	• What is most profitable to suppliers may not be what is most in the interests of consumers; since neither consumers nor suppliers may be very clear about what is in the former's interests, suppliers are allowed a wide range of discretion. • Priorities are determined by the extent to which consumers can be induced to part with their money, and by the costs of satisfying the pattern of "demand."	• Personal professional dedication and public-spirited motivation are likely to be eroded and degenerate into cynicism if others who do not share these feelings are seen as doing well for themselves through blatantly self-seeking behavior. • Priorities are determined by what gives the greatest professional satisfaction.

continued

TABLE 6-3 *Continued*

System Element	Private Systems	Public Systems
	• The profit motive generates a strong incentive toward market segmentation, price discrimination, and tie-in agreements with other professionals.	• Because cost-effectiveness is not accepted as a proper medical responsibility, such pressures merely generate tension between the "professionals" and "managers."
Adjustment mechanism(s)	• Professional ethical rules are used to make overt competition difficult.	• Public systems do not need elaborate cost data for billing purposes and thus do not routinely generate much useful information on costs.
	• Insured consumers who are denied information about quality and competence may collude with doctors (against the insurance carriers) in inflating costs.	• Clinicians know little about costs and have no direct incentive to act on such cost information as they may have; sometimes they may even have disincentives (i.e., cutting costs may make life more difficult or less rewarding for them).
	• Entry into the profession is made difficult and the number of practitioners restricted to maintain profitability.	• Little is known about the relative cost-effectiveness of different treatments; where some information exists, doctors are wary of acting on it until a general professional consensus emerges.
	• If demand for services falls, doctors extend the range of their activities and push out neighboring disciplines.	• It is difficult to phase out facilities that have become redundant because such an action often threatens the livelihood of some concentrated, specialized group; in addition, the people dependent on the facility can be identified, whereas the beneficiaries are dispersed and can only be identified as "statistics."
Success criteria	• Consumers will judge the system by their ability to get someone to do what they need	• Because life expectancy is the easiest aspect of health status to measure, mortality

continued

TABLE 6-3 *Continued*

System Element	Private Systems	Public Systems
Success criteria—*cont'd*	done without making them "medically indigent" or changing their risk rating too adversely.	data and mortality risks predominate in outcomes measurement, to the detriment of assessment of treatments concerned with non-life-threatening situations.
	• Producers will judge the system by how substantial a living they can make through it.	• In the absence of accurate data on cost-effectiveness, producers judge the system by the extent to which it enables them to carry out the treatments that they find most exciting and satisfying.

SOURCE: Based on A. Williams, "Priority Setting in Public and Private Health Care: A Guide Through the Ideological Jungle," *Journal of Health Economics* 7:173-183, 1988.

fully. Those trying to reform the American system are probably in the first position, and those trying to reform the British system are in the second.

If health care reforms in Britain are to succeed—and succeed without abandoning the system's egalitarian ideology—a way must be found to "micromanage" clinicians more effectively. The best hope for doing this appears to lie in convincing doctors that it is their public and professional duty to carry out the policies that have been established by their health authorities; their acceptance of this responsibility in turn depends on the outcome of a much wider struggle for the hearts and minds of the citizenry. The policy dialogue in the media has been vigorous in the United Kingdom, raising hopes that the public will not only come to accept the need for prioritization (there are signs that they may have accepted it already) but also that they will be able to move on to the much more difficult task of agreeing on the broad principles on which such prioritization (i.e., rationing) should be based. The health care system of the future in Britain is likely to be one that in substance will be close to the maximization of equity-weighted quality-adjusted life years (although the public debate is unlikely to be conducted in such abstruse terms). Consensus as to the precise values that go into such a system will probably never be reached— any more than consensus has been achieved in Britain with respect to educational policy, or defense policy, or transport policy. But merely to have health care prioritization a topic of continuous dialogue in the public arena, and subject to continuous review in the light of that dialogue, constitutes an important breakthrough. The entire exercise should greatly strengthen both public maturity and political accountability, which are essential to the democratic management of care and capacity in a national health service in which priorities are based on need.

7

The Meeting of the Twain: Managing Health Care Capital, Capacity, and Costs in Canada

Morris L. Barer and Robert G. Evans

The Canadian and American health care systems differ in three fundamental structural respects: entitlement, management, and environment. Fundamental philosophical differences in the two societies have their outcomes in the different approaches to, and results of, extending entitlement to benefits to their respective populations. The most obvious result distinguishing the two systems is that 30 to 40 million Americans have no health insurance coverage; many millions more have inadequate coverage. The managerial differences reveal themselves in the quite different "targets" of management. In Canada, the targets have largely been at the "macro" level, or systemwide; in the United States, they have been at the "micro" level, in the form of particular clinical interventions, or at the "mini" level, in the form of specific organizational and financial constructs (e.g., health maintenance organizations) intended to manage care patterns for particular subsets of the population. Differences in environment are found in other sectors of the two nations' economies, the interests of which must be balanced against the activities of and benefits from the health care system. In particular, Canada does not have a major industry that develops new technologies with health care applications. Nor is there an informed, articulate private constituency for cost containment, because private employer-based health insurance is vestigial in Canada.

Although these differences have resulted in dramatically different cost experiences (Evans, 1986; Evans et al., 1991) and some clear differences in patterns of health care utilization, this paper argues that the problems of health care system management in both countries are now, and will increasingly become, tied to the management of health care capital: human (particularly physicians), physical (facilities and equipment), and technological (know-how). Such management will require considerable political will on both sides of the border. To date, Canada has been somewhat more successful, largely because of its quite different funding process, but also because those responsible for making major capital decisions are less hampered by competing priorities than their American counterparts.

This discussion begins by elaborating briefly on the fundamental differences (noted above) between the two systems. It then outlines Canada's approach to health care system management, the relationship of that management to the management of each type of health care capital, and the interconnectedness of the three classes of capital. The paper closes with observations on the likely future direction of strategies for health care system management in Canada, on the challenges ahead, and on the significance of some of those challenges for U.S. health care system reform.

WHAT MAKES CANADIAN HEALTH CARE DIFFERENT?

One of the great ironies in the predicament in which health care in the United States finds itself today is that universal coverage or entitlement to benefits—a key to health care system management (and cost control) in Canada and most other Western industrialized countries—is seen in the United States as an elusive target because of its alleged cost-expanding implications. Experience elsewhere continues to suggest that overall (as distinct from public) health care cost control in the absence of some form of universality is impossible. Yet universality, while apparently widely supported by Americans (Blendon and Taylor, 1989), remains elusive because of the perception that achieving it will further increase costs in what is already the world's most expensive health care system. Such cost increases, in contrast to the broadening of coverage, find favor with only a very narrow and clearly identified group of Americans—the "vendors" of services.

The reconciliation of this apparent contradiction is relatively straightforward. Universal coverage for medically necessary services is necessary, but not sufficient, for health care cost control. Extending coverage may increase costs in the United States if it is achieved through "fill-in" coverage, that is, through the addition of more pieces to the jigsaw puzzle of American health care financing. Hospitals operating at relatively low levels of occupancy may be able to raise those rates. But as Wennberg (in this volume) points out, where capacity is relatively fully deployed already (as is presumably the case for physician services), the extension of coverage may have minimal effects on overall use.[1] It may, however, put significant upward pressure on prices. So those in the United States who are concerned about the cost-expanding implications of extending coverage may well be right. But they will be right only because partisans of "autonomy," "pluralism," and "taxation anti-bodies"[2] have used these approaches with almost religious fervor to suppress more comprehensive proposals for health care system reform and, at least so far, have restricted the policy choices to continued "disjointed incrementalism" (Kinzer, 1990).[3]

Within this policy straitjacket, extending coverage to those Americans who are presently uninsured or underinsured would achieve universality but would almost certainly increase health care costs in the United States quite dramatically. Universality is not sufficient to achieve cost control. Whereas those countries with universal coverage have managed to control their health care costs relative to the United States, it has not been the universality per se that has achieved such control. One could quite easily imagine circumstances in Canada that would allow the entire population to be covered for medically necessary hospital and medical care, yet that would produce a cost experience more closely paralleling that of the United States. In fact, during subperiods of the two decades of universal hospital and medical coverage in Canada, some individual provinces have done rather well in mimicking the American cost experience (Barer and Evans, 1986; Hughes, 1991).

Yet universality elsewhere has left American health care costs in a league of their own (Abel-Smith, 1985; Schieber and Poullier, 1991). In what sense is it necessary? In addition to being an objective worth pursuing

---

[1] In fact, this limited effect was precisely what was found when universal health insurance was introduced in Quebec in 1970 (Enterline et al., 1973). The distribution of beneficiaries changed—use by lower income persons increased and use by higher income individuals decreased—but overall use was unchanged.

[2] Thus, for example, one finds the Health Insurance Association of America going to great lengths to highlight the huge tax burden for Americans implied by the adoption of a Canadian-style system. Malignant neglect of the countervailing side of the ledger, the private out-of-pocket costs and private insurance premiums that would be "saved" (but which in some proportion constitute the incomes of members of that association), creates a predictable and highly misleading picture (Neuschler, 1990).

[3] Never mind that systems structured around universal entitlement, such as that of Canada, have, according to the record to date, provided far more autonomy for physicians than has the increasingly clinically managed American system, or that the Canadian system provides at least as much autonomy for the patient in choosing a practitioner and that most Americans seem dissatisfied with the plurality of health insurance schemes. In the heat of the rhetorical debate, the precise nature of the "autonomy" or "pluralism," apparently so coveted, rarely emerges. Nor is it often made explicit which segments of the American population so value these alleged characteristics of the present U.S. "system."

in its own right for reasons of equity and altruism, universality is also a means to a management end. It appears to be necessary to the achievement of cost control because it provides the enabling management structure for such control. Cost experiences in different countries, or in different provinces, states, or regions, reflect the extent to which those responsible for managing health care systems avail themselves of the management opportunities provided by each particular form of universal coverage. And that, in turn, depends on the shifting balance of political influence between vendors and payers.

In Canada, the federal legislation that established the hospital and medical care insurance programs provided grant and tax point transfers to the provinces that were conditional on universality and the establishment of provincial, nonprofit, publicly administered insurance programs to provide coverage for medical and hospital costs. Responsibility for plan management rests with each province, but the broad terms and conditions, at least until now, have been largely dictated by federal fiscal powers.

Thus, in the Canadian context, it is the manner in which universality evolved that has shaped the form of health care management. Unlike the United Kingdom, Canada chose to establish a collection of social insurance programs while leaving the actual provision of care largely in the hands of private "autonomous" medical practitioners. Although most hospitals are public institutions and are funded globally out of public funds, the clinical management of the patients treated in them is a matter left to private practitioners with privileges at each facility. The administration of each institution is handled by an executive staff employed by independent hospital boards.

This does not mean, however, that care is not "managed." Health care in Canada is "macromanaged": provinces manage the financing of the system that provides the care, and that financial management affects the volume and mix of care provided. But the management, at least to date, has been one step removed from the bedside or the clinician's office. "Managed care," even in a broad sense, has come to be associated with a particular set of activities that have gained favor recently in the United States (chart review, outcomes management, development and application of clinical practice guidelines, volume performance standards, second opinion programs, and the like). All of these have the explicit intent of involving more than the attending physician in the micromanagement of patterns of care provided to individual patients. These forms of managed care are explicitly about changing the fundamental nature of the doctor-patient relationship. But they are not the only means available for managing care.

The importance of viewing the American and Canadian systems as occupying different positions along a management continuum cannot be overstated. Too often the debate over system reform in the United States casts

Canada as the system that "rations,"[4] in contrast to the United States, where care is "managed." Such a contrast is, of course, pure rhetorical nonsense. Both (all) systems "ration" (Hadorn and Brook, 1991), but they approach rationing in different ways. Each system chooses to manage the utilization of health care resources differently. The increasingly dominant American approach is to have third parties involved in the physician's microenvironment, to have someone attempt to look over the physician's shoulder and push his or her elbow. The Canadian approach has been to attempt to constrain the macroenvironment, the total size of the health care pie, and to assign (implicitly) the responsibility for micromanagement to those eating it.

In Canada, at least until quite recently, the micromanagement levers have been left largely untouched. Nothing in principle prevents such activity in the Canadian system, although in practice there are powerful political constraints. Certain approaches, however, such as the development of quality assurance programs and physician peer assessment programs (McAuley et al., 1990) appear to be emerging as a new growth industry in Canadian health care. As suggested later, however, they seem to come with more circumscribed and more realistic objectives than are found in the United States; there, managed care appears increasingly (at least to these authors) to be expected to carry the burden of system cost control along with the more micro objectives of improving the effectiveness and efficiency of clinical management of particular health problems. Based on the record to date, its achievements at either level seem underwhelming.

The third fundamental structural difference between Canadian and American health care can be found in the environmental contexts in which each system operates. A significant and economically important share of American productive activity (and capacity) is to be found in technological research, development, sales, and distribution. Much of this activity (e.g., the development and marketing of new pharmaceutical products, of imaging and laser technologies, of orthotics and prostheses) has the American health care system as one of its major potential markets. More use of its products by the health care system means a more profitable technology sector (not to mention a more prosperous group of health care providers). Thus, the dynamic of growth in the health care sector is intertwined with that of these other "derived-demand" sectors. In the current environment, however, the two sectors create competing political imperatives, and the policy problems

---

[4]A leading example of this attitude was the 1989 letter sent over the signature of Alan Nelson, then president of the American Medical Association (AMA), to all AMA members, cautioning that a "Canadian-style health care system could cause rationing of medical services."

that this fundamental conflict poses are characteristics of the American system that are largely absent in the Canadian.[5]

In this context, it is worth noting that if newly developed technologies were to produce cost savings when applied in the health care sector, part of the political problem of competing priorities (health care cost control versus support for technological research and development) would disappear. But the cost savings on one side of the ledger are still income losses on the other; the incentives for the health care system to pick up such technologies are not obvious. It comes as no surprise, then, that the health care industry has a voracious but selective appetite; cost-enhancing technologies are preferred.

This latter point is no less true in Canada than in the United States. The difference is that Canadian politicians do not have to confront these conflicting political objectives to anywhere near the same extent. The development of new pharmaceuticals, medical devices, and the like in Canada represents a minute industry when set against the health care complex. Political initiatives to control health care costs in Canada do not come up against the kind of need that exists in the United States to support and nurture another major set of economic activities.[6] The world of technological innovation in medicine will carry on (and in all likelihood continue to prosper) regardless of what Canada does in the way of health care management. Indeed, the future of the technological development sector in Canada is tied more closely to world markets than to the Canadian health care system.

This knowledge may raise questions about the extent to which Canada's relative cost control success is simply due to the absence of a domestic industrial complex selling to the health care industry. Here, the experience of other countries may inform the discussion. The United Kingdom falls somewhere between Canada and the United States in this respect. It has a major international pharmaceutical presence, whose interests conflict with

---

[5]The military analogy is pervasive here. Not only do some of the technological advances in health care emerge from research that is, in the first instance, militarily motivated, but the military and the health care sectors in the United States share a common current political problem. Both are under intense cost-control pressure, which conflicts with the interests of the complementary technology development sectors for which the military, on the one hand, and the health care sector, on the other, are the major markets.

[6]Canadian policy, however, may be powerfully influenced by the priorities of the American technology industries. The Canadian federal government's Bill C-22, passed in 1987, significantly extended the patent protection of new pharmaceuticals and thereby undercut (probably destroyed) nearly two decades of carefully crafted cost-control policy at the federal and provincial levels. The action was a direct response to American pressure applied at the highest political level.

that of the National Health Service in minimizing the cost of pharmaceuticals, at least for Britons. The pharmaceutical manufacturing sector appears to survive and prosper; in addition, health care there represents significantly less of all productive activity than in Canada. Germany is more like the United States than Canada in this respect, having major pharmaceutical, imaging, and other "high-tech" interests; yet its health care cost experience is more like that of Canada. A rational strategy for all of these countries is to promote the export side of domestic technological industries (especially exports to the United States) while attempting to limit their applications in domestic health care markets. In the United States, however, the domestic health care system represents the largest potential market for the new products. Furthermore, it is a market eager to adopt new innovations in "halfway" technologies (Evans, 1984).

Thus, the United States continues to promote progress in health care technology, apparently oblivious to the fact that such promotion is at odds with the rhetoric of health care cost control. This paradox was nowhere more obvious than at the 1990 International Summit on Health Care and the Economy, sponsored by the University of Texas Health Science Center just prior to the meeting of the G7 countries in Houston. The keynote speakers, Robert Mosbacher and Denton Cooley, both gave inspirational addresses. Unfortunately, the two fundamental messages could not have been more opposed. U.S. Secretary of Commerce Mosbacher opened the summit by emphasizing the need to extend coverage and improve the efficiency with which health care is provided to Americans. He emphasized that uncontrolled health care costs were now a serious drag on American prosperity and economic growth. Cooley, on the other hand, celebrated the glories of modern medicine and extolled the economic virtues of the export potential of the products and services developed and offered by the Texas medical complex (the largest such complex in the country) as a major countercyclical stabilizer for the Houston economy. Unfortunately, neither speaker heard the other (nor, one suspects, would it have mattered if they had).

SO HOW *DOES* CANADA DO IT?

Managing Operations

A considerable literature describing the organization and financing of Canadian health care already exists (see, e.g., Evans, 1984, 1988; Iglehart, 1986a,b; Barer et al., 1988; Evans et al., 1989). Its fundamental characteristics are well known, and any comprehensive attempt at description would detract from the intent of the present paper. In brief outline, each province has its own medical and hospital insurance program, but all adhere to requirements set out in federal legislation. A fundamental element of these programs is that coverage must be offered to the entire population, under uniform terms and conditions. Although a few provinces continue to charge premiums for medical care (in British Columbia, for example, premium revenue represented slightly more than 50 percent of total Medical Services Plan outlays, including the costs of administering the plan, during fiscal 1988–1989), care cannot be denied because of premium payments that are in arrears.

The medical and hospital sectors are financed almost entirely from general revenues (from provincial sources and federal transfers to provinces). In fact, with the enactment in 1984 of the Canada Health Act, "user charges," "extra-billing," and other out-of-pocket medical or hospital costs to patients were largely eliminated because the legislation stipulates dollar-for-dollar reductions in federal cash transfers against any such private charges. In effect, a province that allows such charges asks its population to pay twice, a compelling political deterrent. Not surprisingly, taxation rates are high. On the other hand, private insurance cannot operate in competition with the public medical and hospital programs. With very few exceptions, Canadians do not pay out-of-pocket charges or premiums for these services. Because total health care costs are lower, the savings in private costs outweigh the extra tax payments.

Provincial governments are responsible for the allocative decisions within the health care sector in each province and have a key role to play in the "pricing" of services. Here, the discussion is restricted to medical and hospital care. Most physicians in each province are paid fees for service on the basis of a provincewide fee schedule. Overall average changes in the schedule are periodically negotiated between provincial ministries of health and provincial medical associations (there are separate general practitioner and specialist associations in Quebec). The medical associations determine the internal allocation of these increments. Each fee schedule is associated with a set of payment rules that govern the frequency and circumstances under which particular billed items will be reimbursed. As a result of increasing internal pressure, a number of provincial medical associations have recently begun to develop relative value scales that would remove some of the alleged inequities,[7] but there is no sign of any movement toward a consistent national relative value scale. Although fee experiences in different provinces and during different periods have varied, sometimes dramatically (Barer and Evans, 1986; Hughes, 1991), overall, the process of

---

[7]Much of the internal conflict is over relative incomes, in that procedural specialists have gained some considerable ground over their nonprocedural peers and over general practitioners. This conflict tends to be played out on the fee schedule playing field, despite the fact that those at the lower end of the income distribution have, in fact, fared relatively well on the internal fee allocations (Barer et al., 1992).

bilateral negotiations has held fee increases at, or slightly below, general rates of inflation over the past decade. This process is a key component of managing the Canadian health care system, and it has implications for the management of care (as distinct from costs; Barer et al., 1988). Physician fees have grown much more rapidly in the United States than in Canada; utilization per capita has grown somewhat more rapidly in Canada.

An increasing number of physicians are being paid salaries or are being compensated on a sessional basis, and it appears that most provinces would like to see this trend continue. To date, however, these alternative forms of payment represent a relatively small proportion of total provincial outlays for medical services.

Against this payment backdrop, the supply of physicians in Canada has increased at rates well in excess of population growth for almost 40 years. Estimates to 1990 suggest a population/physician ratio of about 450:1 in Canada; this figure is closer to 400:1 in the United States (Evans et al., 1991). The aggregate income expectations this sustained increase represents, and the growing recognition that fee controls alone do not control costs, have led a number of provinces to introduce so-called macro cost-management techniques (Lomas et al., 1989). Negotiations in most provinces now have utilization "on the table" (over the protests of the medical associations), and some medical associations appear to be willing to give up fee increases to avoid utilization or expenditure caps.

There are a rich variety of capping models. A capped reimbursement agreement could provide for quarterly monitoring of global utilization, with fees in subsequent quarters being temporarily rolled back from schedule values so that expenditures remain within the cap. All variants allow utilization increases for general population growth; some provide additional utilization room for structural population changes or other factors; some involve the sharing of overages between the profession and the provincial ministry of health (Lomas et al., 1989). Finally, individual general practitioner income ceilings have been in place in Quebec for a number of years (Contandriopoulos, 1986; Barer et al., 1988; Lomas et al., 1989), in conjunction with overall expenditure caps.

As noted earlier, funding for hospitals also comes largely from ministry of health budgets. (Only one province still retains hospital insurance premiums.) Salaries and wages of most hospital workers are negotiated on a provincewide basis, between the unions and associations representing the hospital employers. The hospitals, in turn, negotiate annual operating budgets[8] with the ministry of health. Historically these negotiations have been

---

[8]Operating and capital costs are funded differently, although mainly from the same source. Capital costs are addressed in the next section.

rooted rather firmly in the experience of prior years, with some adjustments for new programs. An emerging trend in some ministries of health is the development of more sophisticated population-based funding formulae for hospitals, which take account of the age, sex, and even ethnic structure of the population.

Current consideration by provincial authorities of population-based funding formulae, however, goes beyond the funding of hospitals. There has been a spate of provincial Royal Commission reports in recent years, all of which have recommended some form of regional funding and management (see, e.g., the 1989 report by the Nova Scotia Royal Commission on Health Care and the 1991 report of the British Columbia Royal Commission on Health Care and Costs). But the political pressures against such a policy continue, so far, to thwart any initiatives. One province (Nova Scotia) has already announced that it will not adopt its commission's regionalization recommendations; to date, others have not been that explicit. Ontario is commissioning work that is intended to develop regional funding formulae (Birch and Chambers, 1990), and recent Quebec proposals would allocate medical budgets regionally (Ministère de la Santé et des Services Sociaux, 1990). It seems likely that regional management structures will be developed in Canadian provinces over the next half-decade, in part because provincial ministries of health recognize the inherent logic of population-based funding. Those same ministries, however, may also recognize the advantages of deflecting the centralized political heat that results from attempts to control costs.

Managing Capital

The long-run viability of these Canadian approaches to managing health care costs will depend critically on the will and ability of Canadian policymakers to manage health care capital, including new technology. Health care capital comes in three basic forms: physical (bricks, mortar, machines and equipment), human (health care personnel), and intangible (research and development activities; Barer and Evans, 1990). All share the characteristic that resource commitments at a point in time are intended to generate a future stream of benefits; all correspondingly require the sacrifice of current consumption.

Yet the anticipated stream of future benefits is not the only future effect of today's commitments. Health care capital also creates a future stream of pressures for additional, complementary capital and operating commitments. It is this fundamental characteristic of health care capital that poses the major challenge for the macromanagement of the Canadian health care system and, seen from this side of the border, poses an even greater challenge for the management of health care in the United States.

This intertemporal and interclass capital interdependence is nowhere more evident than in the relationship between physical and human capital. "New non-human capital brings with it demands for, or expectations of, new and often quite specialized *human* capital. Once the human capital is in place, idling physical capital offers the prospect not only of turning off switches on machines, but the redeployment, or costly re-tooling, of the complementary human resources. Not only is the physical capital the raison d'etre for the human resources, but the reverse also becomes true in practice" (Barer and Evans, 1990). New imaging technologies demanded by hospitals that want to remain up to date create derived demands for physicians with the skills and knowledge to manage them. Once the medical care team is in place, a new set of political constituents renders the job of shutting down the capacity (even if it is determined to be obsolete or ineffective) that much more difficult. But this dynamic works equally in the opposite direction. New, highly specialized physicians create derived demands for the complementary "tools of their trade." If fewer cardiac surgeons are trained, there will be fewer coronary artery bypass graft units. Once the units are in place, however, a demand for, among others, perfusionists is created.

The interdependence of the less tangible intellectual capital with the other two classes is no less real. New imaging or laser therapeutic techniques give rise to a host of new forms of physical capital and create derived demands for ever more highly specialized technicians and physicians. The explosion of clinical and technological knowledge makes mastery of any part of it increasingly difficult and creates continuous pressures for subspecialization as a knowledge-control mechanism. In addition, human capital creates demands for itself. New subspecialists covet academic programs through which they can funnel residents to assist with the clinical work. Educational programs tend to be supported not on the basis of whether the products of the programs are required by the population but rather on the basis of the needs of the training institutions and their faculty (Barer and Stoddart, 1991).

The expansionary dynamic of health care capital has roots in the explosion of the physician supply in North America and Europe over the past three decades (Schroeder, 1984; Viefhues, 1988; Evans et al., 1991). Not only do new physicians create demands for new complementary treatment space (hospital beds and other facilities) and technology (their diagnostic and therapeutic arsenal), but they play critical roles in the creation of new knowledge and techniques through their roles in research and development. Although Canada's current per-capita supply of physicians is not as "rich" as that in some European countries (Germany, France), and is actually somewhat lower than that in the United States, it is still widely regarded (at least in Canada) as in excess of desirable levels.

Canada's management of its health care capital has been, like its over-all system management, largely at the macro level. It has not been particularly successful in managing its health care human capital because, unlike most physical capital, human capital is mobile. Each province is accountable for health care spending within its jurisdiction and can more or less successfully control overall levels of funding and the proliferation and diffusion of physical capital. No individual province, however, has control over the supply of physicians who wish to practice in that province (and who submit claims to the provincial plan).

The key to control of physician supply rests with individual medical schools. Yet individual schools will argue (correctly) that reducing their training capacity will have no necessary effect on provincial supply, both because of interprovincial movements of physicians trained in Canada and because of in-migration of foreign medical graduates. There are two paradoxes in these arguments. First, although the logic holds for each school, it does not hold in the aggregate. Yet medical schools in Canada (as in the United States) have shown no inclination to provide collective leadership on this issue. Second, the two dominant problems, to which a continued influx of foreign medical graduates is the solution, are geographic maldistribution of physicians and the service requirements of postgraduate training programs. Domestic solutions to both would again require leadership from the medical schools, which has, to date, not been forthcoming (Barer and Stoddart, 1991).

The problem of interprovincial mobility is felt most acutely in British Columbia. In the mid-1980s, that province attempted to address its particular problems with physician supply growth by limiting the number of physicians who could submit claims for payment to the medical plan. At the end of a rather tortuous legal evolution (Barer, 1988), this policy was overturned on constitutional grounds. Despite some doubt about whether the B.C. Court of Appeals judgment was consistent with prior and subsequent constitutional decisions (Lepofsky, 1989), no other province has yet tested the legality of this approach. In any case, a policy of limiting the number of physicians billing the system would have a clear effect in the implementing province but would make little sense if all provinces did it.

First-year enrollments at Canadian medical schools have declined about 6 percent over the past 7 years (although applications per place have not), and there are increasing pressures for further reductions. The pressures come, rather predictably, from provincial ministries of health, which are responsible for meeting, or otherwise dealing with, the financial pressures created by the burgeoning supply. In contrast, despite the fact that the number of graduates peaked in 1985, no reduction has been seen in the overall number of funded post-M.D. training positions or even in the number of such positions funded by provincial ministries of health (Association of Canadian Medical Colleges, 1990). This may reflect in part the lengthening of requirements in some programs. It seems equally likely, however, that the expansion in post-M.D. positions is increasingly driven by the self-generated "need" for students of ever-growing numbers of residency programs (Barer and Stoddart, 1991).

Canada has not, then, to date, adequately addressed the issue of human capital management. Relative to the United States, however, it has better managed the proliferation of subspecialties. The Royal College of Physicians and Surgeons of Canada recognizes for certification about one-half the number of specialties recognized in the United States. The ratio of general practitioners to specialists in Canada is about 55:45. This management of specialty supply is achieved through ministry of health funding of the vast majority of post-M.D. training positions. Each new residency implies a requirement of from 4 to 6 new funded positions, because a position is necessary for each year of the training. The financial implications of such requirements are not trivial.

Nevertheless, given the downstream income expectations (and the demands for complementary capital) associated with each new specialist, as well as the growing divergence between undergraduate training capacity and post-M.D. funded positions, the management record here seems no more worthy of envy than that on overall supply. Some reductions are anticipated in the size of the post-M.D. training establishment in Canada over the next 5 years, despite a move toward a common 2-year post-M.D. training requirement that would be recognized by all provincial licensing authorities. This expectation may remain unmet if reductions in training capacity will idle, or force the redeployment of, medical school human and physical capital. The threat of such reductions mobilizes powerful, determined opposition. Such opposition historically has been quite successful, because the distribution of losses is much more concentrated (and identifiable) than is the distribution of benefits from downsizing capacity.

As for Canada's management of physical capital, the record is relatively good. Institutional capital (new facilities and beds, new capital equipment) is funded largely through the same provincial ministries of health (with regional districts picking up most of the rest of the costs), although the specifics of approval and allocation vary across provinces (Deber et al., 1988; Bayne and Walker, 1989).[9] Relatively speaking, this process has resulted in an ample supply of hospital beds (which are, in fact, more frequently occupied in Canada than in the United States [Evans, 1990]). But this supply (particularly of acute care beds) has not increased in recent

---

[9]The interested reader will find a relatively detailed description of this process in British Columbia in Barer and Evans (1990).

years to match the growing supply of physicians (Barer and Evans, 1986). Because these two forms of capital are complementary, this asymmetry creates continuous political pressure through physician claims of system underfunding, "shortages," and "waiting lists."

The Canadian centralized process of capital approval, however, has limited the diffusion of diagnostic and therapeutic technology. Because physicians cannot generally receive lump-sum or fee-based funding for capital acquisitions, much of Canada's high-tech capacity is restricted to public hospitals. In turn, all hospitals in each province must go through provincial, and often regional, approval processes that provide at least the potential for rational planning of the acquisition of such equipment. The hospital- and physician-based pressures to have every conceivable piece of new equipment at every hospital are similar to those in the United States. But the diffusion outcomes, the rates of utilization, and the implications for overall hospital costs are quite different in Canada (Detsky et al., 1983, 1990; Rublee, 1989).

Even when hospitals manage to raise local funds for a CT (computed tomography) scanner, for example, the provincial ministry of health is under no obligation to provide the necessary operating funds. In such a case, the hospital must reallocate monies from within its global operating budget or raise the operating funds as well. Taking the former route runs the risk of raising questions within the ministry about how the hospital found the necessary "slack" in a budget about which it is constantly complaining. Although hospitals are raising money for capital expenditures with increasing frequency, such situations remain the exception.

As noted earlier, Canada plays a minor role (on a world scale) in the development of medical technological capital. Most of it simply arrives at the border. Canada has not controlled access to new knowledge—in fact, how could it? Instead, in the manner described above, the macro approach to health care management controls the number of "embodiments" of that new knowledge in new machinery. To date, as suggested above, the record is mixed. How successful Canada has been depends on where one sits, and on one's perception of the value of more, relative to lesser amounts, of different types of health care capital. Some American observers find much to envy in the Canadian approach (Marmor et al., 1990). Others argue that the limitations on the availability of new high tech capital in Canada are a serious drawback to the Canadian system; to support their contention, these observers point to the alleged flow of Canadians in search of high-tech interventions south of the border or to long waiting lists for high-tech interventions. No one suggests that the management process is perfect (Iglehart, 1990). Every health care system is a dynamic set of solutions to the continuing emergence of a series of connected and complex problems. The choice of a health care management approach is a choice among alternative sets.

FROM MACRO- TO MICROMANAGEMENT AND BACK AGAIN?

Largely absent until recently within this macromanaged system has been micro- or clinical management. Provincial ministries of health generally have been more or less content to manage overall costs and the allocation of funds. Although decisions have been made about the availability and location of new technology, those decisions have been based more on financial and political factors than on effectiveness or efficiency evidence. There has been virtually nothing that looks or feels like "managed care," as it is understood in the United States.

Whether this is better or worse than other alternatives, and whether Canada should (as it appears now to be doing) put more energy into micromanagement initiatives (e.g., technology evaluation, continuing competence programs for physicians), depends on the goals of technology and system management. New technologies offer a variety of cost and outcome possibilities, but there are few instances in which information on these possibilities is known in advance of application. For the rest, policymakers must attempt to acquire it after the technologies are put into use, all the while hoping that they (and the population to which they are accountable) do not get too badly "burned" while the evidence accumulates. (Of course, in many cases the evidence never accumulates, but management decisions must still be made.)

Interventions (including any new approach to clinical diagnosis or therapy) may have one of several effects:

a. reduce health care costs while improving or leaving unaltered the health status of recipient patients;

b. increase health care costs but produce substantial and unequivocal improvements in the functional capabilities of recipients;

c. increase health care costs and produce small, positive, often difficult-to-measure increments in the health status of some segments of the patient population;[10] or

d. whatever their costs, produce no or negative effects on health status.

Health care managers in any system should welcome all possible occurrences of type (a) interventions.[11] The management of type (b) technologies can be assisted by technology evaluation, but care must be taken in generalizing

---

[10]Welch has labeled these the "epsilon effects."

[11]The vendors of services, however, are often less supportive; as emphasized earlier, reduced costs translate into reduced incomes for some vendors. If these vendors are in a position to insist that absence of harm be proven *to their satisfaction* before the new technology is introduced, type (a) changes may be slow in coming.

results from one setting to another, let alone across countries. Furthermore, many evaluations are themselves quite costly.

The primary problems of health care system management do not, however, come from type (a) and (b) interventions. Most of the micromanagement (and research) efforts are intended to identify and eliminate type (d) technologies—indeed, they have no place in any health care system. The great danger in this approach is that a single-minded preoccupation with type (d) interventions may skew the application of management energy out of all proportion to their relative importance. Category (c) may be more important quantitatively than the other three categories combined. Moreover, clinical ingenuity and technological progress are likely to ensure a growing stream of such interventions (Wennberg, 1990).

Although category (c) interventions produce small benefits for individual patients, collectively, the high costs of the health gains they offer may swamp the benefits. Heroic measures for the late-stage Alzheimer's disease patient come to mind as an example of a situation in which extremely costly interventions may extend life for a few hours, days, or even weeks (Callahan, 1987). Most people, if they were given the choice at earlier stages in their lives, would choose a different process for the final stage of life.[12] But a person may not have that choice, because new technologies continue to make more things possible and because they are there they will be used.

The problem with many category (c) interventions is that the ethical imperatives within the health care sector make it exceedingly difficult, if not impossible, to make choices against such "epsilon interventions." Cost-effectiveness evidence is unlikely to be available to the management process, because many of these everyday interventions are not individually important enough to warrant the use of limited evaluation research resources. The only practical way to reduce the occurrence of category (c) interventions is to reduce the capital and capacity that makes them possible.

How does Canada manage category (c) and (d) interventions? There seems to be little doubt that Canada lags behind the United States in identifying category (d) technologies. As noted earlier, the macromanagement approach has provided few management incentives, and in fact powerful political disincentives, to look over the clinician's shoulder. Some evidence suggests that Canada has better addressed the epsilon problem within

---

[12]There are, in fact, two conceptually distinct issues here. Life extension per se does not necessarily represent improvement in health status. The person concerned might feel, and genuinely be, "better off dead." An intervention that appears to belong in category (c) when measured only by life expectancy may actually fall into class (d). However, even for "authentic" class (c) interventions, the relation of benefit to cost may be such that a representative individual, looking forward in life, might reasonably judge that he or she would prefer to forego the possibility of such interventions.

the hospital sector than has the United States (Detsky et al., 1983, 1990; Barer and Evans, 1986; Anderson et al., 1989). But it may be less successful in other areas—for example, by providing more physician services for and institutional care of the elderly. As for high-technology diagnostic equipment, Canada's approach of "controlled technological diffusion" has, at least in relation to the United States, controlled technological diffusion. The jury is still out, however, on whether this has made Canadians better or worse off than their better-endowed American neighbors (Evans et al., 1991).

The American managed care approach to category (d) interventions is able to muster political and financial support because it is identifying and promoting the elimination of unequivocally "bad buys." In comparison, the Canadian macromanagement approach may be coming under increasing political pressure as the social consensus on which it rests is threatened by the asymmetry of information dissemination to the public. Much of what Canadian patients (like their American counterparts) learn about the possible benefits of interventions comes from their vendors, for whom doing better means doing more. The predictable result is a growing public perception of an underfunded health care system, bled white by continual financial cutbacks.

There is no informational counterpart to the provincial financial and managerial roles. Provincial ministries of health are loath to become involved in an organized effort to counter the claims of vendors because they fear that they cannot possibly succeed—that they will be perceived as simply projecting a message consistent with their responsibility to control costs, without much regard for outcomes. The research and policy analysis community, which might be expected to assume this role, is too small and, more fundamentally, with few exceptions does not yet see this as a legitimate or appropriate task (Lomas, 1990).

At the same time, the number of "promotional" voices continues to grow far more rapidly than the population, and more rapidly than the real rate of economic growth of the country. Canada, as has been mentioned, has done little to manage its human health capital in a manner consistent with its approach to health care system management. Continued tight control over hospital capacity and over medical care budgets, in the face of a rapidly expanding physician supply, offers very few possible outcomes. That of "loosening the public purse strings" seems unlikely and, on current evidence, unjustifiable. That of forcing physician incomes down, perhaps precipitously, would be politically hazardous, and not necessarily fair to the large majority of the profession. Yet those are the two stark options. They ensure a continuing climate of public conflict.

There is, in fact, a third option, favored by many vendors. The constant pressure of the human capital who depend on an ever-expanding health care system for their own survival and prosperity frequently produces renewed calls for the introduction of private-sector funding. As Iglehart (1990) noted recently, Canada is alone in the Western world in its "resistance to private funding." User fees, in various forms, are an idea that continues to surface, even in Canada. They are proposed regularly by the medical profession, allegedly as a means of reducing cost pressures. In reality, they are seen by the profession as a means to increase expenditures, while reducing public cost pressures.

Nor are vendors the only advocates of greater expenditures through direct access to patients' private resources. It appears that a growing number of relatively well-off Canadians are becoming convinced by the vendors' arguments that public funding cannot or will not support ready access to first-class care for themselves and their families. They are realizing that a limited schedule of user fees will give them an advantage: preference for services, and thus first call on the public funds that will always form the backbone of any health care system.[13] In the end, the funds all come from the same source; thus far, Canadian governments have recognized this and stood by the principle of universal access on equal terms and conditions.

Yet this, too, may be about to change. Recent federal legislation in Canada (Bill C-69) will dramatically reduce the federal contributions intended for provincial health care. The bill froze such contributions for a period of 2 years, and this freeze has recently been extended so that it will now be in place until 1995. The legislation was introduced and passed with surprisingly little fanfare or outcry, either from federal opposition parties or from the provinces, under the cover of a major (and continuing) constitutional crisis. Given historical, federal all-party support for the Canadian medical and hospital insurance programs, the relative silence from the opposition parties suggests that they have not yet fully recognized the potential ramifications of the bill. The glue that holds the system together, that ensures adherence to a common set of principles by all provincial plans, is the federal fiscal role. As that erodes, as the contributions from the federal government become less important, provinces are more likely to go their own ways. In the end, it may be the federal government itself, rather than the medical profession, that drives the wedge of private funding into the door. In the process, however, it may destroy the whole system, a possibility clearly recognized by the profession in its public opposition to Bill C-69. In the view of these authors, this legislation represents a major threat to the Canadian system of financing health care, a threat perpetrated by a federal government increasingly seen by Canadians as slowly disemboweling Canada. The implications for the possibility of macromanagement of

---

[13]This statement includes the American system, in which the rhetoric of private funding obscures the major public role in subsidizing and regulating the "private" system.

health care in Canada are not good. Nevertheless, whatever system (or country) emerges over the longer term, the need for such management will not disappear.

THE FUTURE OF HEALTH CARE MANAGEMENT IN CANADA

Despite these looming dark clouds, macromanagement is likely to continue to dominate the Canadian health care economy for the foreseeable future. But nothing inherent in the Canadian approach guarantees efficiency or effectiveness in the use of health care resources. The outcome—of what gets done, to whom, where, by whom, with what complementary resources, and with what effects—is not necessarily, or even likely to be, the outcome that one might observe if one were able "objectively" to rank all possible interventions and then allocate resources to them up to the current global expenditure ceilings. Macromanagement may be crucial to global cost control, but it is not sufficient to produce the patterns of care sought by micromanagement initiatives.

Canada's record with macromanagement, if viewed from the perspective of cost control, is quite good in comparison to the United States, but unimpressive in comparison to any other country. To a large extent, the current condition of the health care economy is a product of medical education and funding decisions (capital commitments) made in the late 1960s and early 1970s. The demographic projections on which those medical school enrollment decisions were based were made in the early 1960s; it has been known for nearly 20 years that they were grossly in error (too high by about 35 percent by 1991; Barer and Stoddart, 1991). But capital commitment is politically far easier than capital contraction. The incentives to encourage adjustment in the face of new demographic information simply were not in place.

Macromanagement in Canada over the next decade may begin to look more like that in the United Kingdom, as budgeting and management responsibilities are decentralized. But the challenges for smaller managerial units will be no less daunting than those presently faced by the centralized provincial authorities—unless those authorities are willing at the same time to make some hard capital decisions that cannot be made locally.

Yet what of micromanagement? It is at best misleading, at worst dishonest, to promote the notion that micromanagement, if only there was enough of it, would achieve macrocontrol. As Wennberg (1990) has noted, "The inventive nature of the medical mind, the endless possibilities for plausible theories, and the urge all physicians feel to work for and be helpful to their patients combine to make it impossible for outcomes research to keep up with the flow of new medical ideas" (p. 1204). Grumbach and Bodenheimer (1990) describe this phenomenon as the "continual attempt [by physicians] to extend the borders of the medical pasture" (p. 121). Micromanaged care will continue to change the shape and composition of the health care pie; it is unlikely, however, to have much effect on its size. In this, it seems remarkably (and depressingly) similar to basic medical research. In that sphere, as each "insulting" organism is identified and a clinical assault mounted, three others emerge.[14] Continued uncertainty about the specifics of appropriate care seems likely to hinder the effort for some time to come (Grumbach and Bodenheimer, 1990).

Clinical management in Canada is the object of increasing interest and effort, but resources are not being channeled into this arena because of a belief that it will replace the need for macromanagement. Rather, outcomes research, the development of clinical practice guidelines, clinical competence assurance activities, and the like are seen in the Canadian context as tools for guiding resource allocation and organization within global budgets—not as replacements for those budgets. No amount of micromanagement or outcomes research can tell a society how much of its scarce real resources should be devoted to health care. There will always be more interventions that produce "epsilon effects" than can possibly be evaluated.[15]

A commitment to maintaining a system of global budgets still leaves the problem of setting and controlling them. The present Canadian approach of bilateral negotiation and, in the end and if necessary, imposition may not be sustainable politically in the absence of new policy directions for capital management. A reduction in the rate of production of new physicians seems an essential starting point. But even that simple step will require a new, heretofore elusive, national consensus. Physicians are a national resource, budgets a provincial responsibility. The elements pushing stakeholders toward such a consensus may now be there: the present fiscal climate, a growing understanding of the broader (non-health-care) determinants of population health (Evans and Stoddart, 1990), the increasing range of questions raised by research on outcomes and procedural variations regarding the population benefits of ever-larger allocations of limited public funds to health care (Roos and Roos, 1990), and a common sense of political fatigue from the prospect of having to manage an ever-larger medical community. The hope is that these elements will finally come together

---

[14]Opportunistic infections of AIDS patients offer the clearest example of this phenomenon. As the patient's T-cell count progressively declines, new infections gain a foothold. Increasing research efforts find new treatments for each, which are effective only until the count falls sufficiently to bring on the next infection.

[15]What is transpiring in the United States suggests that micromanagement is being saddled with a far more onerous burden. Outcomes research and managed care appear to be the replacement for the lost promise of, first, more regulation and, then, more competition (which was, in fact, more regulation in a different package) as vehicles of cost control.

in Canada to produce a new contractionist era in medical resource policy. It will not have come a year too soon.

REFERENCES

Abel-Smith, B. 1985. Who is the odd man out: The experience of Western Europe in containing the costs of health care. *Milbank Memorial Fund Quarterly* 63:1-17.

Anderson, G. M., Newhouse, J. P., and Roos, L. L. 1989. Hospital care for elderly patients with diseases of the circulatory system: A comparison of hospital use in the United States and Canada. *New England Journal of Medicine* 321:1443-1448.

Association of Canadian Medical Colleges. 1990. *Canadian Medical Education Statistics 1990.* Ottawa: The Association.

Barer, M. L. 1988. Regulating physician supply: The evolution of British Columbia's Bill 41. *Journal of Health Politics, Policy and Law* 13:1-25.

Barer, M. L., and Evans, R. G. 1986. Riding north on a south-bound horse? Expenditures, prices, utilization and incomes in the Canadian health care system. In: R. G. Evans and G. L. Stoddart, eds. *Medicare at Maturity: Achievements, Lessons and Challenges.* Calgary: University of Calgary Press, pp. 53-163.

Barer, M. L., and Evans, R. G. 1990. *Reflections on the Financing of Hospital Capital: A Canadian Perspective.* HPRU Paper No. 90:17D. Vancouver: University of British Columbia, Health Policy Research Unit, Division of Health Services Research and Development.

Barer, M. L., and Stoddart, G. L. 1991. *Toward Integrated Medical Resource Policies for Canada: Background Document.* Discussion Paper 91:6D, Centre for Health Services and Policy Research, University of British Columbia; and Working Paper 91-7, Centre for Health Economics and Policy Analysis, McMaster University.

Barer, M. L., Evans, R. G., and Labelle, R. 1988. Fee controls as cost control: Tales from the frozen north. *Milbank Quarterly* 66:1-64.

Barer, M. L., Evans, R. G., and Haazen, D. S. 1992. The effects of medical care policy in British Columbia: Utilization trends in the 1980s. In: R. Deber and G. Thompson, eds. *Restructuring Canada's Health Services System: How Do We Get There From Here?* Toronto: University of Toronto Press, pp. 13-17.

Bayne, L., and Walker, M. 1989. *Capital Equipment Acquisition: A Discussion Paper.* Vancouver: Stevenson Kellogg Ernst and Whinney.

Birch, S., and Chambers, S. 1990. Development and application of a needs-based methodology for allocating health-care resources among populations at the county level. Unpublished mimeo. Hamilton: McMaster University, Centre for Health Economics and Policy Analysis.

Blendon, R. J., and Taylor, H. 1989. Views on health care: Public opinion in three nations. *Health Affairs* 8:149-157.

British Columbia, Royal Commission on Health Care and Costs. 1991. *Closer to Home.* Vol. 2, *Report.* Victoria, B.C.: Crown Publishers.

Callahan, D. 1987. *Setting Limits: Medical Goals in an Aging Society.* New York: Simon and Schuster.

Contandriopoulos, A.-P. 1986. Cost containment through payment mechanisms: The Quebec experience. *Journal of Public Health Policy* 72:224-238.

Deber, R. B., Thompson, G. G., and Leatt, P. 1988. Technology acquisition in Canada: Control in a regulated market. *International Journal of Technology Assessment in Health Care* 4:185-206.

Detsky, A. S., Stacey, S. R., and Bombardier, C. 1983. The effectiveness of a regulatory strategy in containing hospital costs: The Ontario experience, 1967-1981. *New England Journal of Medicine* 309:151-159.

Detsky, A. S., O'Rourke, K., Naylor, C. D., Stacey, S. R., and Kitchens, J. M. 1990. Containing Ontario's hospital costs under universal insurance in the 1980s: What was the record? *Canadian Medical Association Journal* 142:565-572.

Enterline, P. E., Salter, V., McDonald, A. D., McDonald, J. C. 1973. The distribution of medical services before and after "free" medical care—the Quebec experience. *New England Journal of Medicine* 289:1174-1178.

Evans, R. G. 1984. *Strained Mercy: The Economics of Canadian Health Care*. Toronto: Butterworths.

Evans, R. G. 1986. Finding the levers, finding the courage: Lessons from cost containment in North America. *Journal of Health Politics, Policy and Law* 11:585-616.

Evans, R. G. 1988. "We'll take care of it for you": Health care in the Canadian community. *Daedalus* 117:155-189.

Evans, R. G. 1990. Accessible, acceptable, and affordable: Financing health care in Canada. In: *Improving Access to Affordable Health Care*. The Richard and Hinda Rosenthal Lectures. Washington, D.C.: Institute of Medicine, pp. 7-47.

Evans, R. G., and Stoddart, G. L. 1990. Producing health, consuming health care. *Social Science and Medicine* 31(12):1347-1363.

Evans, R. G., Lomas, J., Barer, M. L., Labelle, R. J., Fooks, C., Stoddart, G. L., et al. 1989. Controlling health expenditures—the Canadian reality. *New England Journal of Medicine* 320:571-577.

Evans, R. G., Barer, M. L., and Hertzman, C. 1991. The twenty year experiment: Accounting for, explaining, and evaluating health care cost containment in Canada and the United States. In: G. S. Omenn, J. E. Fielding, and L. B. Lave, eds. *Annual Review of Public Health*, Vol. 12. Palo Alto, Calif.: Annual Reviews, Inc., pp. 481-518.

Grumbach, K., and Bodenheimer, T. 1990. Reins or fences: A physician's view of cost containment. *Health Affairs* 9(4):120-126.

Hadorn, D. C., and Brook, R. H. 1991. The health care resource allocation debate: Defining our terms. Paper presented at the conference, "Creating a Fair and Reasonable Basic Benefit Plan Using Clinical Guidelines," sponsored by the California Public Employees' Retirement System's Health Benefits Advisory Council, Sacramento, California, April 24-26.

Hughes, J. S. 1991. How well has Canada contained the costs of doctoring? *Journal of the American Medical Association* 265:2347-2351.

Iglehart, J. K. 1986a. Canada's health care system (Part 1). *New England Journal of Medicine* 315:202-208.

Iglehart, J. K. 1986b. Canada's health care system (Part 2). *New England Journal of Medicine* 315:778-784.

Iglehart, J. K. 1990. Canada's health care system faces its problems. *New England Journal of Medicine* 322:562-568.

Kinzer, D. M. 1990. Universal entitlement to health care: Can we get there from here? *New England Journal of Medicine* 322:467-470.

Lepofsky, M. D. 1989. A problematic judicial foray into legislative policy-making: Wilson v. B.C. Medical Services Commission. *Canadian Bar Review* 68:614-629.

Lomas, J. 1990. Finding audiences, changing beliefs: The structure of research use in Canadian health policy. *Journal of Health Politics, Policy and Law* 15:525-542.

Lomas, J., Fooks, C., Rice, T., and Labelle, R. J. 1989. Paying physicians in Canada: Minding our Ps and Qs. *Health Affairs* 8(1):80-102.

Marmor, T. R., Mashaw, J. L., and Harvey, P. L. 1990. *America's Misunderstood Welfare State: Persistent Myths, Enduring Realities*. New York: Basic Books.

McAuley, R. G., Paul, W. M., Morrison, G. H., Beckett, R. F., and Goldsmith, C. H. 1990.

Five-year results of the peer assessment program of the College of Physicians and Surgeons of Ontario. *Canadian Medical Association Journal* 143:1193-1199.

Ministère de la Santé et des Services Sociaux. 1990. Une Réforme Axée Sur Le Citoyen. Quebec City.

Neuschler, E. 1990. *Canadian Health Care: The Implications of Public Health Insurance.* Research Bulletin. Washington, D.C.: Health Insurance Association of America.

Nova Scotia, Royal Commission on Health Care. 1989. *Towards a New Strategy* (report). Halifax, N.S.: The Queen's Printer for Nova Scotia.

Roos, N. P., and Roos, L. L. 1990. *Limiting Medicine.* Document No. 17B. Toronto: Program in Population Health, Canadian Institute for Advanced Research.

Rublee, D. A. 1989. Medical technology in Canada, Germany, and the United States. *Health Affairs* 8(3):178-181.

Schieber, G. J., and Poullier, J.-P. 1991. International health spending: Issues and trends. *Health Affairs* 10(Spring):106-116.

Schroeder, S. 1984. Western European responses to physician oversupply. *Journal of the American Medical Association* 252:373-384.

Viefhues, H., ed. 1988. *Medical Manpower in the European Community.* New York: Springer-Verlag.

Wennberg, J. E. 1990. Outcomes research, cost containment, and the fear of health care rationing. *New England Journal of Medicine* 323:1202-1204.

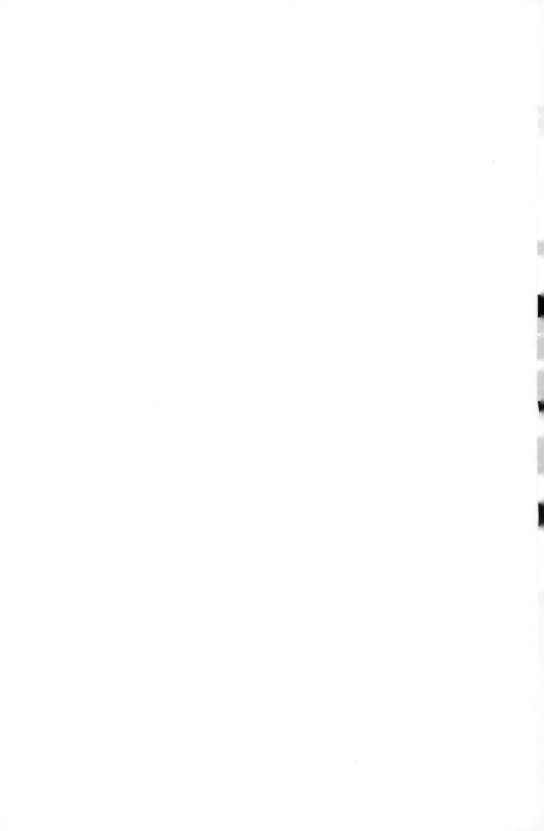

Part IV
Implications for Providers

8

New Technology Adoption in the Hospital

Paul F. Griner

Medical technology adoption decisions in hospitals may occur through planned acquisitions or through uncontrolled changes in medical practice. They reflect a complex set of dynamics, with method of reimbursement being only one, albeit an important one, of those forces. These dynamics must be understood before there can be any hope of developing optimal approaches to the adoption of new technology.

This paper first presents a working definition of new technology, followed by a discussion of the various factors that influence decisions regarding its adoption. The reader should bear in mind that these factors are described from the perspective of a hospital physician administrator. This perspective reflects a mixture of knowledge of the benefits and limits of technology on the one hand and awareness of its drawing power on the other. The discussion includes selected data related to the effect of these factors on patterns of technology adoption. The paper closes with several predictions for the future as a way of focusing and stimulating debate.

NEW TECHNOLOGY: WHAT ARE ITS COMPONENTS?

New technology may be arbitrarily classified into five groups:

1. new diagnostic or therapeutic equipment, such as linear accelerators;
2. expensive procedures—for example, transplantation;

3. pharmaceuticals—the fastest-growing segment of the hospital economy, comprising such subareas as biologics developed through genetic engineering and expensive antibiotics;

4. "supportive" technology—examples are hospital information systems and intensive care unit monitors; and

5. "hidden" new technology—changes in medical practice as a result of new knowledge that causes a hospital's existing technology, both diagnostic and therapeutic, to be applied in new ways.

The last category of new technology represents unplanned changes in the day-to-day life of hospital practice that often have significant cost implications but that generally do not come to light until after the change has been in place for a period of time. Some examples are the use of magnetic resonance imaging (MRI) to evaluate the internal structure of the knee and the use of gamma globulin to treat immune disorders of the blood.

FACTORS INFLUENCING THE ADOPTION AND USE OF TECHNOLOGY

Any strategy designed to promote discriminating approaches to the adoption and use of new technology must recognize and take into account the influence of certain factors (Table 8-1). These factors are discussed in the sections below.

Method of Financing

New equipment and hospital renovation (e.g., to accommodate a new program) require capital. The first factor to consider in new technology adoption is thus the hospital's pool of reserves. Does the hospital have the funds needed to renovate space and acquire new equipment? Its endowment, its other sources of nonoperating revenue, and its cash reserves are the primary components of its pool of reserves. The extent of that pool is largely a function of the hospital's ability to generate surpluses from its

TABLE 8-1 Factors Influencing the Adoption of New Technology

1. Method of financing "up-front" costs
2. Method of recovering incremental operating costs, including depreciation
3. Regulation
4. Level of competition
5. Capacity
6. Evidence of effectiveness
7. Hospital/medical staff organizational relationships
8. Decision-making processes

day-to-day operations and to generate nonoperating revenue from gifts and other sources. Operating surpluses, in turn, are largely a function of the level of rate regulation to which a hospital is subject.[1] In the underregulated states of the Midwest, hospital cash reserves tend to be high; reserves of up to $150 million in some of the large midwestern teaching hospitals are not unusual. Conversely, in the heavily regulated hospitals of the Northeast, operating surpluses are uncommon, and for many hospitals (e.g., most New York state hospitals), reserves are nonexistent. Cash for capital expenditures must therefore come from borrowing, and the hospital's borrowing capacity is determined by its overall financial position. It is not surprising, as the data presented later in this discussion show, that new technology is introduced and disseminated more slowly in states that limit capacity through rate regulation.

Recovery of Operating Costs

Financing the initial cost of new technology is one thing; obtaining reimbursement for its operating costs can be quite another. Reimbursement is more complex than financing because there are two important variables involved: the level of regulation and the payers. Among states requiring certificates of need,[2] approval may apply equally to all payers, including health maintenance organizations (HMOs), or just to Medicaid. New York is a good example of a state that requires a certificate of need; as one might imagine, adoption of new technology in this state is more conservative than in any other. Where certification of need is not required, other factors may then assume greater importance.

The ability of the payment system to adapt to changes in the cost of a service may also influence the rate of adoption of new technology. For example, the diagnosis-related group (DRG) system associated with Medicare appears to be a disincentive to the introduction of new technology because the rate of recalibration of DRGs for the incremental cost of the new technology occurs quite slowly (Kane and Manoukian, 1989). In another example, one might anticipate that the problem of fixed-price reimbursement for inpatient care will slow the introduction of some pharmaceuticals, particularly those developed through genetic engineering for highly specific uses at considerable cost.

---

[1]Rate regulation is the payment for care of an individual patient that a regulatory entity allows a hospital to collect. It may be based on a per-diem figure or it may be a fixed payment per admission according to the diagnosis-related group.

[2]In some states, certificate of need regulation requires that hospitals justify the need for a capital project (e.g., device, facility, or program) on the basis of community or regional need.

An additional aspect of recovering the cost of new technology is recovery of the cost of the initial investment, that is, capital cost recovery through depreciation, which should be distinguished from recovery of operating costs. By and large, regardless of the method of reimbursement, capital costs traditionally have been passed on to payers and reimbursed fully. This is likely to change, however, given the proposal by the U.S. Health Care Financing Administration (HCFA) to incorporate capital expenditures into the DRG-based reimbursement per diagnostic category. Although this approach may help control costs overall, it has no mechanism to account for the legitimate capital costs of individual hospitals and is causing much concern among hospital administrators.

Data are available to support these observations bearing on the relationship of capital reserves, operating surpluses, and regulation on the one hand and adoption of new technology on the other. There are 30 teaching hospitals in the states of New York, Massachusetts, Connecticut, and New Jersey, where hospital reimbursement is heavily regulated. The average operating margin of these hospitals in 1989 was –$2.4 million, compared with an operating surplus averaging $6 million for the country's remaining teaching hospitals (Fishman et al., 1990). In addition, annual capital expenditures for building improvements and equipment replacement, reasonable surrogates for overall capital outlays, were 25 percent less for the 30 Northeast hospitals than such expenditures for similar hospitals throughout the rest of the country.

Comparing upstate versus downstate New York hospitals reveals another factor that may influence the adoption of new technology, namely, the hospital's share of service to the poor. New York metropolitan hospitals had operating deficits in 1989 (–3.2 percent) that were 60 percent higher than their upstate counterparts (–2.0 percent). This difference in part reflected more charity services by downstate hospitals and bad debt levels that were twice as high as levels for upstate hospitals (6 percent versus 3 percent, respectively). It is little wonder that New York City hospitals frequently complain of their inability to compete for new technology (Fishman et al., 1990).

Regulatory Equity

Fueled by technological advances and stimulated by reimbursement incentives, much health care that previously involved hospitalization is now provided in ambulatory settings. What one might refer to as unbalanced regulation—less regulatory oversight than is required for hospitals—has provided a further stimulus for the rapid growth of out-of-hospital technology (e.g., ambulatory surgical centers, imaging centers, ambulatory rehabilitation centers). In many areas of the country, hospitals that wish to expand their ambulatory services are at a disadvantage because of unbalanced certificate of need requirements compared with outpatient facilities. Such facilities contribute significantly to the rate of inflation in Part B Medicare, a rate that is rising more than twice as fast as that of hospitals. This is an area that demands more regulatory attention.

Level of Competition

The level of competition among hospitals in a region is an important determinant in the adoption of new technology, particularly in areas with excess hospital capacity. This phenomenon occurs most often in regions with little regulatory control of capacity but with substantial growth in the use of managed care. Examples of such areas include Minneapolis, Chicago, and California.

Where competition is great, the principal focus of the hospital administrator becomes the hospital's market share. High-technology services tend to attract patients, and the more services a hospital can offer, the more competitive it will be for exclusive contracts with employers and other third-party payers. Such circumstances support a tendency to develop duplicate services considerably in excess of regional needs. As a result, managed care models do not appear to be as effective as regulation in controlling the adoption of new technology. (The closed-panel Kaiser system may be an exception to this generalization because, in this form of managed care, both the hospital and its medical staff have incentives to acquire and use technology sparingly.) Few data are available to prove or disprove this hypothesis, although some information bearing on the number of hospital FTEs (full-time-equivalent employees) according to the reimbursement environment may be acceptable as a surrogate, given that even new technology tends to be labor intensive. Fishman and colleagues (1990) present figures for the number of FTEs per occupied hospital bed, after adjusting for case mix, in four heavily regulated northeastern states, four underregulated midwestern states, and two states with a sizable proportion of managed care. The number of FTEs per bed in these regions are 5.2, 6.1, and 6.9, respectively. These data support the hypothesis that in the field of health care, regulation is more effective than competition in controlling costs.

Worth sharing in regard to this issue are the experiences of the author and his colleagues (Block et al., 1987) during the 1980s in Rochester, New York, under an experimental hospital payment system. This payment program encompassed two extremes. One featured a community cap on capital expenditures; that is, all major capital projects required review and approval by the hospital coalition before subsequent review by the local health systems agency and the state. During the period 1980 through 1987, the oper-

TABLE 8-2   Rochester Hospital's Experimental Program Under Two
Systems

Effect	Global Budget (1985-1987)	All-Payer Diagnosis-Related Group (1988–1990)
Revenue	Predictable (pro); variably adequate (con)	Variable; determined by volume and case mix
Community health care costs	Controlled	Unpredictable; inflationary
Incentive	Manage services	Obtain market share
Introduction of new technology	Controlled (pro); rationed (con)	Available to all (pro); inflationary (con)
Incentive for ambulatory alternatives to inpatient care	Yes	No
Physician satisfaction	±	+
Access to hospital services	+	++
Quality of care	Good	Good
Cooperative spirit	Good	Constrained

ating expenses of the participating hospitals were guaranteed but capped
under a global budget, providing a ceiling on both operating and capital
costs. In the other extreme of the payment system (1988–1990) the hospitals functioned under an all-payer DRG system and capital costs were not
limited.

Table 8-2 displays the advantages and disadvantages of these two systems. Under the system of capped operating and capital budgets (i.e., the
Global Budget column), revenue was predictable and hospital costs were
controlled. From 1980 through 1987, hospital costs increased by 168 percent nationwide; in Rochester, the increase was 108 percent. The average
Blue Cross premium in the United States in 1989 was $3,500; in Rochester,
it was $1,600. Managers spent most of their time managing, new technolo-
gy was introduced in a controlled fashion, incentives for ambulatory alternatives to hospitalization were great, and adequate markers existed to con-
firm that quality of care was good. Some physicians felt that access to
hospital or high-technology services was being constrained, and hospital
boards were concerned about the loss of sovereignty. These observations,
in combination with a year when demands (and costs) of hospital services
outstripped the dollars available, led to an interest in exploring the opposite
alternative. Consequently, from 1988 through 1990, the hospitals were
reimbursed under an all-payer DRG system with a capital pass-through.

Physicians were more satisfied, access was probably better, hospital boards were happier, and revenues increased at a higher rate; but community health care costs were higher, managers spent most of their time trying to gain market share (despite the observation that the rate of bed occupancy was high for all hospitals), considerable duplication of new technology occurred, and incentives for ambulatory alternatives to inpatient care virtually disappeared.

The experience in Rochester is a classic example of the conflict between the need to address the collective interests of society on the one hand and the interests of the individual on the other (the individual in this case being the patient, the physician, and the hospital all together). One system favored the greater social good; the other favored the individual. The goal must be a balanced approach that recognizes both needs. Ultimately, some combination of local, state, and federal regulation, together with price-driven competition, should promote that balance.

Table 8-3 presents some data that reflect major differences in the introduction of new technology throughout the country, according to whether regulation or competition prevails (Fishman et al., 1990). The four heavily regulated states mentioned earlier (New York, New Jersey, Connecticut, and Massachusetts) are compared with the country at large in terms of the proportion of institutions that perform various transplant procedures and another procedure (cochlear implants) whose efficacy remains to be determined. Striking differences are apparent. Two-thirds of the less regulated teaching hospitals perform bone marrow transplants, but only one-quarter of similar hospitals in the heavily regulated states undertake the procedure. The proportion of teaching hospitals that perform heart transplants in less regulated states is 4.5 times the proportion of hospitals performing them in the more regulated states (78 percent versus 17 percent, respectively). If one focuses only on those less regulated states in which managed care has a

TABLE 8-3   Proportion of Hospitals Performing Selected Procedures According to Level of Regulation

Procedure	More Regulated (% of hospitals)	Less Regulated (% of hospitals)
Transplant		
Adrenal	0	8
Bone marrow	27	66
Heart	17	78
Liver	17	45
Cochlear implant	7	40

significant effect on patterns of practice (i.e., California and Minnesota), these differences appear to hold up. These data support the conclusion that strategies designed to limit overall capacity are more effective than competitive strategies, including managed care, in controlling the introduction of new technology.

Other Factors That Influence the Adoption of New Technology

The four factors discussed above—method of financing a technology's initial cost, method of recovering operating costs, level of regulation, and degree of competition—are the principal factors influencing the decisions of hospital administrators regarding the adoption of new technology. There are a number of others as well, the hospital's capacity for technology assessment being one. Some hospitals (e.g., Johns Hopkins) have an office of technology assessment, which requires medical staff to support initiatives for new technology with evidence of scientific efficacy before other considerations are explored. At Strong Memorial Hospital in Rochester, New York, more than $1 million was saved over 4 years through the application of a protocol that restricted the use of tissue plasminogen activator (t-PA) to patients for whom streptokinase was not appropriate. The protocol was developed by a process of consensus among interested faculty after reviewing the relevant literature on the subject. Such decisions, which are not without political risk, require the medical staff to accept responsibility for prudent use of the hospital's resources.

Hospital-medical staff organizational relationships are yet another factor bearing on the adoption of new technology. Until recently, the hospital has been expected to provide all of the resources needed for its medical staff to deliver patient care. But as the availability of hospital capital decreases, interesting financial relationships are developing in some instances between hospitals and medical staff. Some examples are joint ventures for the acquisition of and operation of new technology, or arrangements whereby staff members purchase equipment and are responsible for its operating costs, while the hospital advances money for working capital, applying standard banking practices for its repayment.

The locus of decision making in the hospital is becoming an important aspect of new technology adoption decisions. The ultimate responsibility for policy rests with the hospital board. In cases in which hospital boards exercise that authority, the adoption of new technology is determined largely by affordability. In instances in which hospital boards still serve in a pro forma mode, medical staff pressures may override financial reality testing and local or regional needs. Finally, in many teaching hospitals, the research activities of faculty lead to the development and introduction of new diagnostic and therapeutic technology.

Hidden New Technology

So-called hidden new technology refers to changes in the application of technology in hospital practice, which occur almost daily and which often have significant cost implications. Such changes occur in an unplanned way and result from the generation and dissemination of new knowledge bearing on clinical diagnosis and management (e.g., new applications of MRI, new uses of existing expensive pharmaceuticals such as gammaglobulin for the treatment of immunologic disorders). The pharmacy budget of Strong Memorial Hospital in Rochester, New York, has increased by 75 percent in fewer than 5 years. Across the country, hospital pharmacy budgets are the fastest growing segment of the hospital economy. Because of these trends, hospitals are beginning to put in place more comprehensive drug surveillance systems to monitor changes in medical practice and to ensure that these new practices adhere to reasonable standards of cost-effectiveness.

Hidden technology encompasses many other aspects of the day-to-day care of hospitalized patients. Changes in automatic infusion pumps, hospital beds, cancer chemotherapy protocols, monitors/defibrillators, and pulse oximeters are but a few of the many enhancements to care that are introduced daily throughout the hospital, usually without a management master plan.

SUMMARY

The following sums up a combination of facts and the author's personal experience regarding the adoption of new technology.

1. New technology is introduced more slowly in areas of the country in which health facilities are heavily regulated than areas in which competitive strategies are promoted.

2. A regional capital expenditures cap tied to a global operating budget appears to be the most effective method of controlling capital costs. The Rochester experience bears this out, although this paper does not include all the supporting data.

3. The single most important determinant of a hospital's adoption of new technology is the hospital's operating margin. This statement holds true both when payment programs are designed to control capacity and when they are designed to stimulate competition.

4. Hospitals are beginning to recognize the many other factors that influence the adoption of new technology—for example, changes in organizational and financial relationships with medical staff, development of in-house technology assessment capabilities, and the increasing role of the hospital's governing body in decisions about major hospital expenditures.

5. Two predictions for the future: one that is already becoming clear is that throughout the 1990s, the adoption of new technology will occur more slowly as hospital operating surpluses continue to fall. The other prediction is that hospitals and their medical staffs will have to develop innovative organizational and financial relationships involving shared risk. These relationships will ensure that the adoption of new technology is the result of a balance between the hospital's competitive desire for excellence and the region's interest in helping to achieve affordability by ensuring that services that are not actually needed are not made available.

REFERENCES

Block, J., Regenstreif, D., and Griner, P. 1987. A community hospital payment experiment outperforms national experience: The hospital experimental payment program in Rochester, NY. *Journal of the American Medical Association* 2:193-197.

Fishman, L. E., Serrin, K. G., and Bigelow, J. S., eds. 1990. *Council of Teaching Hospitals: Survey of Academic Medical Center Hospitals' Financial and General Operating Data, 1989.* Washington, D.C.: Association of American Medical Colleges.

Kane, N. M., and Manoukian, P. D. 1989. The effect of the Medicare prospective payment system on the adoption of new technology: The case for cochlear implants. *New England Journal of Medicine* 20:1378-1383.

9

Physicians' Acquisition and Use of New Technology in an Era of Economic Constraints

Bruce J. Hillman

Physicians perceive a growing harshness in the health care environment. They are concerned that the policy initiatives of the 1980s and the apparent increasing stringency of the coming decade will negatively affect both their ability to deliver what they believe to be optimal care for their patients and their own incomes and enjoyment of medical practice.

Central to these concerns is the access of physicians to medical technology. In prospect, a physician's ability to acquire medical technology depends on the regulatory, reimbursement, and competitive milieus in which he or she practices, as well as on the perceived technical and clinical potentials of the technology. This paper discusses to what extent physicians might be influenced by current health policies and the expected medical organizational environment with respect to their decisions to acquire and use new technologies. The paper focuses specifically on the acquisition of major medical devices, because these technologies have been especially scrutinized by health policy researchers and policy decision makers.

This discussion is composed of three parts. First, in the belief that recent past experience might presage what will occur in the immediate future, the paper presents earlier research describing how physicians responded to environmental influences in deciding whether to acquire a new medical technology of the 1980s—magnetic resonance imaging (MRI). The second part addresses the changes that have occurred since the early diffusion of MRI. The third section considers how these changes might selectively influence physicians who are considering the acquisition of some future new technology.

DIFFUSION OF MAGNETIC RESONANCE IMAGING INTO CLINICAL PRACTICE

This section of the paper discusses research on nonmedical influences that have affected MRI acquisition (Hillman, 1986; Hillman et al., 1986, 1987a,b). During 1984–1985, 3 years after the first MRI scanner was introduced in the United States, investigators at the RAND Corporation studied the diffusion of MRI. Physicians at that time were, as now, concerned about the development of a much more restrictive budgeting environment than they had previously confronted. Prospective payment for hospital inpatient care had just been introduced for Medicare patients, and many states still had vigorous health planning bodies. The Food and Drug Administration (FDA) had designated MRI as a class 3 technology—requiring extensive premarketing tests and approval before general diffusion—and there was virtually no third-party reimbursement for the procedure. The prevailing opinion was that these conditions, partly by the design of policymakers and partly as a result of circumstances, would reinforce the already significant uncertainties surrounding the technology and act as potent disincentives to physicians and other providers that might be considering MRI acquisition.

MRI appeared on the health care scene to proffer important benefits that were not supplied by other technologies: imaging without ionizing radiation or injected or ingested contrast material; improved differentiation of body tissues; and the promise of new types of information concerning metabolism and physiology. Physicians were excited by these possibilities and their potential to benefit patients' health. But there were also major uncertainties: how high the acquisition and operational costs of the technology would be; which version of the technology would become ascendant; where the technology would best be located; and what MRI would add to what could be learned about patients' problems by using already well-understood technologies (e.g., x-ray, computed tomography [CT], ultrasound).

Clearly, many of the uncertainties reflected, in part, a concern that influences external to characteristics of MRI in the health care milieu might restrict potential acquirers of MRI in their ability to successfully operate MRI facilities. To determine to what extent such restrictions were felt, the RAND investigators adopted a case study approach. They performed 83 extended, guided, open-ended interviews with individuals interested in MRI-related issues—manufacturing, selling, regulating, acquiring, and reimbursing. Thirty-seven of the interviews were with potential acquirers of MRI; almost uniformly, these interviews represented physicians' views. This paper explores how regulatory, reimbursement, and competitive influences affected physicians' consideration of MRI acquisition.

Regulation of Magnetic Resonance Imaging Acquisition

Two major regulatory factors were extant during the early diffusion of MRI: the responsibilities of the FDA in approving new medical devices, and health planning, predominantly in the form of state certificate-of-need (CON) activities.

The Food and Drug Administration

MRI was the first major technology to be designated class 3 by the FDA under the 1976 Medical Device Amendments to the Food, Drug, and Cosmetics Act. This classification required MRI manufacturers to submit their devices to rigorous testing to ensure the safety and efficacy of their technology. Rather than evaluate MRI devices as a class of technologies, the FDA decided to consider each manufacturer's device and each alteration of each device separately, portending a very extended process. In principle, prior to obtaining FDA certification, a firm could neither advertise its device nor sell its devices for profit. Facilities were also affected: they were prohibited from charging patients more than their actual costs.

Despite these constraints, marketing proceeded with little interruption. At the time of the RAND study, the FDA had just issued its first premarketing approvals; the devices of most companies had not yet been approved. Nevertheless, the RAND investigations could discern no important differences in the advertising of companies with and without approval. Manufacturers without approval advertised MRI "generically" in medical journals and magazines but made clear their views on characteristics that reflected their own approach to the technology. Corporate "detail" personnel touted real or imagined advantages of their technology vis-à-vis others and promised impending FDA approval and third-party reimbursement. In actuality, FDA approval processes and the decisions on reimbursement from a proliferating number of independent payment entities would require considerable time, and no one could actually predict when they might be concluded.

To develop the data necessary to obtain FDA approval, each manufacturer developed alliances with a number of clinical sites—hospitals and radiologists' practices, for the most part. The manufacturers provided various incentives to physicians to participate in their data-gathering activities, including discounting the price of the MRI scanner or, in some cases, even providing the technology free of charge. Sometimes, because there was virtually no third-party reimbursement for MRI, manufacturers also paid a stipend for performing scans. In other instances, physicians and institutions were designated as test sites even though they provided little data; the RAND team believed these were actually "sales" disguised as premarketing approval activities to circumvent FDA regulations.

Those interviewed by the RAND investigators generally responded quite positively to MRI. Physicians believed that although the FDA approval process clearly would be drawn out, eventually all the devices would achieve approval. The basis for this view related to the charge of the FDA itself. Physicians knew that MRI was safe—there was already considerable experience with the fundamentals of the technology and with patients, both in the United States and elsewhere. The FDA's responsibility for determining efficacy hinges on whether the device does what a manufacturer's labeling claims it will do, which in the case of MRI is to provide images of normal and pathologic anatomy. Again, more than sufficient information was available to potential acquirers that this was the case. Representatives of health maintenance organizations (HMOs) were the only providers interviewed who were more restrained in their enthusiasm for MRI. However, the views of these individuals were more a reflection of corporate fiscal philosophy than any specific concerns related to FDA regulation.

As far as the RAND researchers could determine, concerns over FDA approval inhibited no physician or facility interested in MRI from acquiring the technology. Indeed, the need of manufacturers to establish relationships with providers to obtain premarketing approval may well have enhanced early diffusion.

Certificate-of-Need Regulations[1]

State regulatory statutes, predominantly those involving CONs, had a quite different effect on MRI diffusion, depending on the stringency of a particular state's requirements. CON regulation was empowered by the Health Planning and Resources Development Act of 1974 and was directed particularly at providers to constrain their building of new facilities and their acquisition of major technologies. The act empowered states to establish health systems agencies to administer regulations that the states individually would enact. By the time of the RAND study, shortly after these agencies had been defunded by the Reagan administration, CON administration varied enormously among the states in terms of scope and effectiveness (Salkever and Bice, 1976; Bice and Urban, 1982; Brown, 1983; Steinberg, 1985).

---

[1]CON regulations most particularly affected the ability of hospitals to add facilities or acquire expensive technologies by setting a maximum amount that a hospital could spend without first requesting the permission of the state's health systems agency (by filing a CON application). In all but a very few states, outpatient facilities and physicians' offices were exempt from this process.

To deal efficiently with the variation among the states, the RAND investigators concentrated their efforts in five states that in their view spanned the regulatory spectrum: California and Arizona, which considered themselves "free markets," providing no serious regulatory obstacles to technology acquisition; Illinois and New York, which tightly controlled hospital acquisition of technologies and planned assessments of MRI at a small number of hospitals chosen to receive the technology—but which did not attempt to control the acquisition of scanners in outpatient settings; and Massachusetts, which effectively constrained acquisition of MRI by all providers through a combination of CON (called DON, or determination of need, in Massachusetts) and payment rate regulation. Massachusetts had decided to permit initial acquisition of MRI by only eight hospitals.

In California and Arizona, physicians perceived or actually had no difficulty in obtaining the technology—none, that is, that could be laid to the door of state agencies. A telling observation in the Los Angeles area, where RAND is located, was that one MRI was planned for every mile of a 6-mile stretch of Wilshire Boulevard; by the end of 1985, there were believed to be 25 MRI scanners planned for or operating in Los Angeles and its environs. The motivation for MRI acquisition in California and Arizona was largely competitive and is discussed below.

In Illinois and New York, the intent was to plan hospital acquisition according to the results of assessments of the clinical utility of the device. Initially, relatively few hospitals would be allowed to acquire the technology, and it was to be these few installations that would provide the data for further CON approvals. The states, however, controlled acquisition of the technology by hospitals but not by outpatient facilities, and this quickly led to the hospitals becoming competitively disadvantaged. A further factor was that this development occurred while hospitals were busy accommodating the revenue reductions that accompanied prospective payment under Medicare and the attempts of other payers to reduce cost shifting (i.e., increasing charges to some payers to compensate for reduced payments by others). The confluence of these phenomena put hospitals, the traditional leaders in new technology acquisition, at a serious disadvantage, thus opening a new niche for other prospective providers of MRI services. As a result, the RAND team reported that new entities not previously engaged in providing medical technology services became interested in MRI, and new types of financial arrangements were developed.

With hospitals in states with active CON processes being placed at a disadvantage in terms of acquiring MRI, new sources of capital were needed to finance such acquisitions. The arrangements, which included venture capitalists, health care corporations, and, to a greater extent than in the past, physicians, seemed to be based more on the opportunity for financial gain than on a desire to deliver a medical service. Because of the considerable financial risk posed by acquisition of such an expensive technology, the participants in these arrangements sought to secure enough of a patient base to make the imaging venture successful. Physician investors were recruited on the basis of their ability to refer patients for MRI services, imaging specialists were excluded because they provided no such benefit to the partnership, and there were reports of facilities basing returns on investment on the number of referrals made by the investor.

Providers in Massachusetts understood that to acquire MRI they would have to convince the state that they offered special advantages over other candidates. The state would permit the purchase of relatively few scanners, and the process of selecting those purchasers would be an extended one. Providers thus reasoned that their chances of access to MRI would be enhanced if they went into the CON process along with other providers. Massachusetts was the only state in the RAND study in which consortia were formed to acquire MRI. This pattern existed despite experience with computed tomography scanners suggesting that consortial operations of high technology posed considerable difficulties (Brust et al., 1981).

Regardless of whether a hospital intended to actually operate an MRI facility, it nevertheless filed a CON application, expecting that by the time the process resulted in its selection, perhaps many years hence, it would be ready for the technology. (This trend was observed in hospitals with more than 200 beds.) In essence, filing a CON application was viewed as the means of holding a place in line. This practice, however, imposed an additional burden on an already ponderous and expensive bureaucracy, drawing out the selection process. Indeed, many argued that the cost of the bureaucracy in Massachusetts outweighed the savings of limited diffusion, while providers decried poor patient access to the benefits of MRI. Incontrovertibly, however, whether or not it was to the benefit of the populace, CON was effective in limiting the diffusion of MRI in Massachusetts.

Reimbursement for Magnetic Resonance Imaging

MRI began to diffuse at a time when third-party payers were in the first stages of confronting increasing financial constraints. As noted earlier, the federal government had just instituted prospective payment for Medicare inpatients. In addition, policymakers were discussing whether to institute prospective payment for all physicians or, alternatively, if this proved infeasible, at least for hospital-based physicians. Research was being conducted to evaluate these possibilities (Mitchell, 1985; Ginsburg et al., 1986). Other third-party payers, faced with rising health care expenditures, were considering the adoption of the Medicare initiatives. They were also raising their rates to major benefits purchasers, but at the same time they were under pressure from those purchasers to identify ways to reduce their costs.

On another front, health maintenance organizations were becoming serious competitors, recruiting patients from traditional indemnity insurance plans.

In general, reimbursement agencies viewed MRI suspiciously. It had been less than a decade since they had noted the increased expenditures associated with the introduction of CT scanning; although by this time it was acknowledged that CT had been a beneficial, possibly even cost-effective advance (Banta, 1980; Evens, 1980), the feeling remained that a great deal of waste had accompanied the introduction of the technology. Purchasers seemed aware of the potential benefits of MRI, but most were not convinced that the advances demonstrated to that point were significant enough and different enough from CT to warrant coverage.

At this stage in the diffusion of MRI, there was little scientific evaluation of the technology; what had been published, although considerable, was fraught with biases and dealt in large part with small, selected patient samples (Cooper et al., 1988; Kent and Larson, 1988). A Blue Shield Association assessment—based only on the peer-reviewed literature—indicated that the benefits of MRI were insufficiently proven and recommended against general coverage; MRI proponents argued that the methodology of the study was biased and the findings outmoded. The Health Care Financing Administration (HCFA) began an extended evaluation to determine its coverage policy. Uncertainty remained about how capital reimbursement would be handled under prospective payment.

Interviews conducted by the RAND investigators with prospective acquirers of MRI elicited much concern and anxiety over coming alterations in the reimbursement environment. The technology was more expensive than any previously considered for acquisition--as much as $3 million to purchase and site and up to $800,000 per year to operate. Nonetheless, in no instance did the RAND team find that providers had been dissuaded from acquisition by considerations related to reimbursement. The general belief was that despite what most considered to be "brave talk," resistance to reimbursement on the part of third-party payers was uncoordinated. Payers had never before been able to decline payment for the use of major new technologies, and they were unlikely to be able to do so with MRI. This was particularly true with respect to HCFA; prospective MRI acquirers felt that the agency had delayed too long for it to exercise any option but general coverage. Diffusion and experience with MRI were too extensive and the lay, professional, and corporate pressures favoring coverage for most uses were too powerful to resist.

The RAND researchers found little evidence that either the reimbursement initiatives of the early 1980s or the threat of further impending reimbursement innovations was retarding MRI diffusion. Most of the providers interviewed noted that in the absence of third-party reimbursement, MRI was likely to lose money, at least in the short term. To minimize such losses, acquirers were instituting new payment requirements that they conceded they had never considered in the past, including payment by the patient prior to scanning and reduced "charity" care.

Certain elements of the reimbursement milieu—the uncertainty over how capital reimbursement would be handled under the diagnosis-related group (DRG) system and a reduced ability of hospitals to shift costs— probably promoted early acquisition decisions. (Providers hoped by early acquisition to be "grandfathered" under the old rules.) Concerns over reimbursement probably affected some siting decisions, as well as who would own and operate the devices. As with CON regulation, reimbursement considerations produced a disadvantage with regard to acquisition of technology by hospitals. In concert with the tax advantages favoring for-profit ownership, these issues promoted outpatient siting of MRI.

Competition Over Magnetic Resonance Imaging

The RAND investigators evaluated competition among providers in the same five states in which they had assessed the effects of regulation. In states other than Massachusetts (where, as noted earlier, regulation effectively constrained access to the technology), there was ardent competition over MRI. Three forms of competition can be identified: competition to provide MRI services, competition over patients, and competition among specialties for control of the technology.

The health care policy initiatives of the 1980s were designed, in part, to introduce price competition into medicine. Yet the RAND study team found no instance in which providers considered reducing prices as a means of attracting patients to MRI services. Rather, providers expressed the intention of competing on the basis of the service and developing their marketing efforts more fully than they had ever done before.

The goal of such marketing was to use MRI as a competitive instrument to enhance utilization of a provider's other services. Experiences with CT scanning had given most providers a healthy respect for the power of a new technology to imbue them with a desirable image. Consequently, they viewed MRI as a tool in their battles with local competitors to attract referring physicians, and hence patients, a strategy that would eventually lead to their controlling a larger share of the local market. Their belief was that if they could use MRI to get patients "in the door," they might "capture" them for their other, more remunerative services. A number of early MRI purchasers, who had acquired the technology on this basis, were disappointed when they found that local physicians, concerned over the possible loss of their patients, were reluctant to refer them for scans.

Competition among MRI facilities over referring physicians consequently took a peculiar turn. Given the very high financial risks associated with such an expensive technology, coupled with expected coming financial constraints, facilities vied for the patronage of the physicians most likely to have a high number of potential referrals for MRI scans: neurologists, neurosurgeons, and orthopedists. Frequently, providers offered these physicians special inducements to refer patients to their facilities. Most commonly, the physicians became limited partners in facilities being operated as entrepreneurial ventures or even in joint ventures with hospitals. Despite concerns that such financial involvement might inappropriately influence referrals, lead to abuse of the technology, and infringe on traditional medical ethics (Relman, 1985; Hyman and Williamson, 1989; Morreim, 1989), this practice appeared to be growing rapidly in popularity. (See also the series of letters to the editor and editor's response in the January 23, 1986, issue of *The New England Journal of Medicine* [Vol. 314, No. 4, pp. 250–253].) The competition for physicians and their patients, which was intended to secure a sufficient patient stream to enable financially stable MRI operation, in fact strained traditional relationships among providers and promoted early MRI acquisition.

In addition to competition in providing services and for patients, the RAND researchers observed enhanced competition among specialties over the control of MRI. Turf battles over technology are not new in medicine; this one, however, appeared to be more contentious than previous struggles, possibly because of the high financial and scientific stakes associated with MRI, in concert with physicians' concerns that their ability to sustain their incomes by providing traditional services might be compromised by the more draconian coming milieu. Radiologists, the specialists traditionally responsible for medical imaging, were the earliest and most frequent purchasers of scanners. They were also the physicians who most often advised hospital administrators and were most instrumental in helping to formulate administrators' views. However, radiologists do not primarily care for patients; they depend for referrals on other physicians, which puts them at a disadvantage in the more entrepreneurial context of MRI.

Many of the providers interviewed in the RAND study indicated that they were uncomfortable in proceeding with MRI acquisition but that the competitive environment dictated such an action. Their view was that they gained a competitive advantage by being the first MRI facility in their locale. (Being second meant that fewer of the most desirable referring physicians would be available.) Yet in no instance did the presence of an existing facility dissuade a provider from pursuing MRI acquisition; in these cases, providers cited the existence of other facilities as evidence that if they did not hurry their acquisition, they might be left out entirely. Overall, the RAND investigators concluded that competition among providers was a potent force encouraging the early diffusion of MRI technology.

Summary: The Acquisition of Magnetic Resonance Imaging

From the foregoing, it is evident that physicians—whether representing themselves or an organization—were largely unaffected by the intended thrust of regulatory, reimbursement, and competitive influences in what they themselves believed to be a harsh environment for technology acquisition. Perhaps they simply did not understand the full implications of the policy initiatives opposing MRI purchase. It is likely, however, that physicians' decisions were guided by two considerations: first, although hostile, the forces opposing technology acquisition were still disorganized and were likely, in the end, to be ineffectual; and second, physicians in the past had always found a way to access new technology—MRI would be no different.

The physicians were correct in these surmises. The technology was seductive, and the policies that had been intended to retard its acquisition were ineffective in the face of significant professional and lay demand for MRI.

TECHNOLOGY ACQUISITION IN THE "NEW HEALTH CARE" ERA

There is a general perception among physicians that the times have grown tougher, especially over the past few years. Despite the recent experience with MRI, many observers believe that physicians might be more responsive now to environmental influences opposing technology acquisition than they were in the 1980s. Certainly, imposing barriers have been erected that might well dissuade physicians from purchasing an expensive new technology similar to MRI. But there are also aspects of the milieu that might reasonably encourage acquisition. Table 9-1 lists various aspects of the health care environment that might promote or retard technology acquisition. As the table indicates, several might be expected to have both positive and negative effects. This section considers how particular influences might be expected to affect technology acquisition by physicians in the coming years.

TABLE 9-1 Influences in the Environment That Promote or Retard New Technology Acquisition

Promoting	Retarding
Nature of technology	Nature of technology
Hospitals and regulation	Hospitals and regulation
Competition for patients	Competition for patients
Providers' turf	Providers' turf
	Reimbursement
	Managed care

Nature of Technology

One important aspect of recent technological innovation has been an emphasis on developing technologies that are safer and less invasive. MRI is a good example, as are the development of digital subtraction angiography for outpatient arteriography, ambulatory dialysis, and technological modifications that permit more surgery to be performed on an outpatient basis. In part, the emergence of this trend is related to the realization that medical technologies have an important role in improving the comfort of care and the quality of life, as well as in extending its length. The development of less invasive technology is also a response to the policy environment, which has favored more flexible siting, particularly siting outside of hospitals. That newer technologies are amenable to outpatient siting is likely to continue to encourage their acquisition. Outpatient use of technology is still relatively free of regulatory constraints and enjoys more favorable reimbursement than inpatient use. The high cost of many new technologies is a potential deterrent to their acquisition but, as with MRI, physicians and other entities still find significant incentives for financial investments in outpatient medical services. The sole disincentive in this regard is the recent congressional prohibition against physicians having ownership interests in outpatient laboratory facilities to which they refer patients and the threat that in the future this ban might be extended to other types of medical facilities.

Hospitals and Regulation

Although some states still maintain CON policies, the overall sense is that health planning generally is weakening. Although this trend might have portended the reemergence of hospitals as aggressive early acquirers of new technology, there are few signs of such activities. Indeed, hospitals now appear more financially debilitated than they were even in the previous decade. They remain disadvantaged under current reimbursement policies and are less able to shift costs among payers, given the increasing volumes of contracted and managed care. As a result, there is a persistent, advantageous niche for entrepreneurial technology acquisition in outpatient settings by physicians and other entities, either jointly with or exclusive of hospitals. These potential providers of technologically advanced services still have access to capital, tax incentives, and mechanisms to ensure a sufficient volume of patients—most notably through self-referral—and to encourage new technology acquisition (ECRI Technology Management Assessment, 1985).

Competition for Patients

Physicians' incomes have kept pace with or exceeded inflation over the past decade, despite declining patient rolls (Starr, 1982). This pattern has been largely attributed to increasing intensity of care, fueled in part by the assimilation of technologies into office practice (Holohan and Zuckerman, 1990). Demand by patients for the use of innovative technologies and their appreciation of the convenience of receiving all of their care in their physician's office have further encouraged these trends. New reimbursement policies now seek to reduce payment for technological care but do little to reduce utilization by individual physicians, who often have a financial incentive to continue or even increase the use of technology. A significant counterbalancing influence, however, is that even independent physicians increasingly participate in managed care, either as members of preferred provider organizations or as contractors to HMOs. In this situation, physicians must compete for patients on the basis of price as well as on the services they offer. Presumably, they will have to consider whether the overhead they will assume in purchasing a technology will diminish their price competitiveness.

Reimbursement

A number of recent reimbursement initiatives might be expected, individually and cumulatively, to affect the ability of physicians to acquire and use new technologies profitably. Perhaps the most significant is HCFA's implementation of a resource-based fee schedule for physician payment under Medicare, which replaces the traditional "reasonable, customary, and usual" method. The major avowed intent of this change is to reduce compensation for what HCFA considers overcompensated, technology-based services in favor of more time-intensive activities, such as taking patient histories and performing physical examinations. Other payers also are currently, or are considering, implementing fee schedules with similar goals. In addition, reliance on precertification, fee ceilings, and limits on balance billing is growing and would be expected to influence technology acquisition and use adversely. Capitated payments for bundled care[2] are increasingly popular with HMOs and clearly make the use of technology financially disad-

---

[2]The provider assumes financial risk for the care of patients by accepting a lump sum payment to provide a "unit" of service. This "unit" is often a period of time, such as a year. If the provider spends less on care than the lump sum amount, he or she profits; if more, the provider experiences a financial loss. Thus, under capitation, there is a fiscal disincentive to employ medical technology, particularly if it is deemed to be of marginal benefit.

vantageous. Many physicians fear that if capitation becomes the dominant payment mechanism, as many believe it might in the future, it would inappropriately curtail modern technological medicine.

Since the late 1970s, payers have voiced concerns about whether their outlays for services that require new high-technology devices return consonant benefits in improved health. A central concern is that little assessment of such technology occurs before its general diffusion. Certainly, this was the case with MRI: aside from the studies required for FDA certification, no scientific assessment occurred for at least 5 years after its introduction into the United States, and little has occurred as of today (Cooper et al., 1988; Kent and Larson, 1988). The resultant uncertainties regarding appropriate application generate unnecessary costs in excess capacity, duplicative studies, financially motivated abuse, and early obsolescence. Payers have threatened to tie reimbursement more closely to scientific evidence that using a new technology improves patient health. Efforts in this regard, however, have been uncoordinated, underfunded, and, as in the case of MRI, unsuccessful. In 1989, the federal government established yet another in a line of agencies intended to foster and coordinate technology assessment—the Agency for Health Care Policy and Research (AHCPR). Unlike its predecessors, however, a major focus of AHCPR's activities is the investigation of the outcomes of medical practice; it is expected to advise HCFA on decisions concerning Medicare coverage. Although AHCPR has not received the level of funding that was originally expected or that would be sufficient to address this charge in a serious fashion, there remains an expectation that, to reduce their costs, both private and public payers must soon consider patient outcomes to a greater extent in their coverage deliberations. Should this occur, the period necessary to assess the effectiveness of a new technology and physicians' concerns over eventual reimbursement might be sufficiently great that diffusion would be slowed.

Managed Care

In the article by Wennberg in this volume, a distinction is made between "micromanaged" and "global limits" types of managed care. Currently, in the United States, a continuum of forms of managed care reflect various combinations of aspects of the philosophies of micromanaged care and managed care with global limits. Managed care in some form, including HMOs, preferred provider organizations, and utilization controls, now accounts for nearly 40 percent of the health care market. It is expected to continue to grow—perhaps to encompass as much as 70 percent of the U.S. population. One intent of managed care is to reduce the use of marginal and inappropriate technology. In staff-model HMOs, an example of a global limits approach, this reduction is accomplished in part by queuing and by providing financial and other incentives to member physicians to use the community's technology resources less frequently. The growing success of this type of managed care entity has allowed it to assimilate more technologies into its own operations, which offers tighter internal control of utilization. Virtually all managed care agencies seek to reduce their technology-related outlays by encouraging potential contract providers to competitively discount their fees and by paying for bundled services, such as in capitation arrangements. Indemnity insurers, as well as HMOs, have increasingly relied on micromanagement, including precertification and the development of standardized approaches to clinical presentation, to control what they view as marginal technology utilization. The emphasis of managed care on cost containment presages a more cautious approach to new technology acquisition and utilization in the future.

Providers' Turf

The personal motivations of physicians for acquiring a new technology usually include intellectual enjoyment, the pride associated with being on the "cutting edge," the respect of one's peers, being able to apply the technology to benefit patients, and the possibility of greater financial remuneration (Hillman et al., 1984). The confluence of a number of the factors described in the preceding sections impinges on the issue of which groups of physicians can most benefit from technology acquisition in the current organizational climate and in the expected climate of the future. Financial concerns are particularly acute and increasingly may be the motivation for a physician's acquisition of a particular technology. In 1990, an article in the *Wall Street Journal* entitled "Warm Bodies" described how physicians who previously had referred patients to radiologists for diagnostic imaging studies were now attempting to coerce these same radiologists into "kicking back" a portion of the payments from these referrals. The threat that constituted the coercion, which had materialized in some cases, was that failure to do so would result in the referring physicians' establishing their own facilities (Waldholz and Bogdanich, 1989).

There is ample evidence that ownership of technologies by physicians—particularly when the technologies are located in their offices—engenders a capacity for technology utilization that is almost always exploited. Recent research indicates that office ownership of imaging technologies by nonradiologist physicians results in four times the frequency of imaging utilization compared with physicians who refer their patients to radiologists for similar services (Hillman et al., 1990). The Inspector General's office recently has published "safe harbor guidelines" that define how freestanding facilities may be organized and operated so as not to be legally culpable for conflict of interest. Congress is considering statutes that would further restrict physicians' ownership of freestanding facilities to which they refer patients, but little consideration has been given to the same circumstance in physicians' offices.

HOW MIGHT PHYSICIANS RESPOND TO THE "NEW HEALTH CARE" ENVIRONMENT?

It should be evident from the foregoing that the current and expected future health care environments present physicians with a complex, often interrelated set of considerations that might affect their decisions concerning the acquisition of expensive medical devices. The focus of this paper has been on such devices because they have been highly visible technologies with respect to the attention paid them in the scientific and lay media; they have also served as focuses for policy research and for issues related to reimbursement. It is important to note that the adoption of these technologies probably differs in ways from the adoption of drugs, procedures, and even less expensive devices. Among these differences are the means by which physicians first learn of the new technology, what influences affect the acquisition decision, and characteristics of the key decision makers.

How responsive physicians are to the considerations described in this paper depends, at least in part, on how well these factors coincide with the criteria physicians actually use in making technology acquisition decisions. In this regard, something can be learned from experiences with previous technologies (Greer, 1981; Hillman et al., 1986).

Physicians, in this author's opinion, first consider how the purchase of a new technology might benefit their patients and fulfill their patients' preferences. A related consideration is the specific attributes of the technology and, to a lesser extent, what remains uncertain about it. The characteristics of a physician's practice (e.g., solo, small group, multispecialty group), the costs of the technology (to own and operate), and the kinds of difficulties the technology presents are also important. Note that all of these "primary considerations" are, for the most part, remote from concerns about the status of the general health care environment. Most physicians consider only secondarily (at least consciously) the financial rewards they might generate or how the regulatory, reimbursement, and competitive milieu might affect their ability to operate the technology successfully.

This lack of convergence between the intents of policymakers, payers, and regulatory agencies and physicians' considerations suggests that, at least in the near term, very little may change in how physicians approach acquisition of a new technology. Despite their anxiety over the harshness of the environment at the advent of MRI, physicians behaved as they have always behaved with respect to their acquisition decisions. This "business as usual" attitude is likely to continue until physicians are faced with a failure of this approach. Clearly, the stringency with which regulatory agencies and health care payers approach their cost-containment initiatives will be a major influence on physician responsiveness with regard to technology acquisition and utilization. Nonetheless, the ingenuity shown by providers in circumventing restrictions in the past, and the considerable ambiguity proffered by the current environment, suggest that physicians' technology-related practices may change to a lesser extent than many authorities expect.

REFERENCES

Banta, H. D. 1980. Computed tomography: Cost containment misdirected. *American Journal of Public Health* 70:215-216.

Bice, T. W., and Urban, N. 1982. *Effects of Regulation on the Diffusion of Computed Tomography Scanners*. Grant No. HS03750. Washington, D.C.: National Center for Health Services Research.

Brown, L. D. 1983. Common sense meets implementation: Certificate of need regulation in the states. *Journal of Health Politics, Policy and Law* 8:480-494.

Brust, J. C. M., Dickinson, P. C. T., and Healton, E. B. 1981. Failure of CT sharing in a large municipal hospital. *New England Journal of Medicine* 304:1388-1393.

Cooper, L. S., Chalmers, T. C., McCally, M., Berrier, J., and Sacks, H. S. 1988. The poor quality of early evaluations of MR imaging. *Journal of the American Medical Association* 259:3277-3280.

ECRI Technology Management Assessment. 1985. Meeting the challenge of free standing imaging centers. Options for hospitals and hospital based radiologists. *Journal of Health Care Technology* 1:257-278.

Evens, R. G. 1980. The economics of computed tomography: Comparison with other health care costs. *Radiology* 136:509-510.

Ginsburg, P. B., Newhouse, J. P., Mitchell, J., Palmer, A., Freeman, M., Hillman, B., et al. 1986. *Planning a Demonstration of Per Case Reimbursement for Inpatient Services Under Medicare*. Pub. No. R-378 HCFA. Santa Monica, Calif.: RAND Corporation.

Greer, A. L. 1981. Medical technology: Assessment, adoption and utilization. *Journal of Medical Systems* 5:129-145.

Hillman, B. J. 1986. Government health policy and the diffusion of new medical devices. *Health Services Research* 21:681-711.

Hillman, B. J., Joseph, C. A., Mabry, M. R., Sunshine, J. H., Kennedy, S. D., and Noether, M. 1990. Frequency and costs of diagnostic imaging in office practice—A comparison of self-referring and radiologist-referring physicians. *New England Journal of Medicine* 323:1604-1608.

Hillman, B. J., Neu, C. R., Winkler, J. D., Aroesty, J., Rettig, R. A., and Williams, A. P. 1987a. The diffusion of magnetic resonance imaging scanners in a changing U.S. health care environment. *International Journal of Technology Assessment in Health Care* 3:545-553.

Hillman, B. J., Neu, C. R., Winkler, J. D., Aroesty, J., Rettig, R. A., and Williams, A. P. 1987b. How experiences with x-ray computed tomography influenced providers' plans for magnetic resonance imaging scanners. *International Journal of Technology Assessment in Health Care* 3:554-559.

Hillman, B. J., Neu, C. R., Winkler, J. D., Aroesty, J., Rettig, R. A., and Williams, A. P. 1986.

Diffusion of Magnetic Resonance Imaging into Clinical Practice. Pub. No. R3392-HHS. Santa Monica, Calif.: RAND Corporation.

Hillman, B. J., Winkler, J. D., Phelps, C. E., Aroesty, J., and Williams, A. P. 1984. Adoption and diffusion of a new imaging technology: A magnetic resonance imaging perspective. *American Journal of Radiology* 143:913-917.

Holohan, J., and Zuckerman, S. 1990. Understanding the recent growth in Medicare physician expenditures. *Journal of the American Medical Association* 263:1658-1661.

Hyman, D. A., and Williamson, J. V. 1989. Setting the limits on physicians' entrepreneurship. *New England Journal of Medicine* 320:1275-1277.

Kent, D. L., and Larson, E. B. 1988. Magnetic resonance imaging of the brain and spine. *Annals of Internal Medicine* 108:402-424.

Mitchell, J. B. 1985. Physician DRGs. *New England Journal of Medicine* 313:670-675.

Morreim, E. H. 1989. Conflicts of interest: Profits and problems in physician referrals. *Journal of the American Medical Association* 262:390-394.

Relman, A. S. 1985. Dealing with conflicts of interest. *New England Journal of Medicine* 313:749-751.

Salkever, D. S., and Bice, T. W. 1976. The impact of certificate of need controls on hospital investments. *Milbank Memorial Fund Quarterly* 54:185-214.

Starr, P. 1982. *The Social Transformation of American Medicine.* New York: Basic Books, pp. 420-425.

Steinberg, E. P. 1985. The impact of regulation and payment innovations on acquisition of new imaging technologies. *Radiology Clinics of North America* 23:381-389.

Waldholz, M., and Bogdanich, W. 1989. Warm bodies: Doctor-owned labs earn lavish profits in a captive market. *Wall Street Journal*, March 1, pp. A1, A6.

Part V
Implications for Patients

10

The Patient's Stake in the Changing Health Care Economy

Albert G. Mulley, Jr.

The focus of this volume is the impact of the changing health care economy on technological innovation. The changing economy affects innovation by altering the environment of decision makers—changing their incentives and their perceptions of what is, and will be, valued in health care. Other papers in the volume address such changes from the perspective of health care providers or of those in industry and academia who develop new technologies. The purpose of this paper is to consider the patient's stake in the changing health care economy. Focusing on and fully understanding the patient's perspective can bring a critical advantage, for it is what health care does to and for patients that determines its value.

To understand the health care economy, one must understand the decision-making process that determines consumption of medical services and thereby the allocation of health care resources. Two clinical examples will clarify both the patient's role in decision making and the patient's stake in how decision making is affected by the changing economy. These examples, treatment of low back pain and treatment of breast cancer, involve choices that depend both on professional knowledge and on personal value judgments and preferences. As the discussion shows, serious questions can be raised about the adequacy of the professional knowledge base and about whether treatment decisions accurately reflect the preferences of those who must bear the consequences.

These problems with the adequacy of the knowledge base and the physician's role as the rational agent of the patient in a relationship characterized by extreme asymmetry of information have been blamed for widespread variation in medical practices, which in turn has heightened concerns about the cost and quality of medical care (Wennberg et al., 1982; Mulley, 1990). These failings of the professional model of resource allocation have motivated policymakers to effect changes in the health care economy. The policy solutions have been drawn from two different kinds of models: the market model and various forms of managed decision making, which have been characterized by Friedson as the bureaucratic model (Friedson, 1990; Mulley, 1991). These two models are most evident in policies designed to promote efficiency through competition among providers and through direct management of clinical decision making. Each model implies different roles and responsibilities for doctors, patients, and policymakers. Each also portends different opportunities and constraints for innovators who would bring new drugs, devices, or procedures into use.

Focusing on what is at stake for patients brings one to the conclusion that objective information is critical not only to good decision making, and thereby resource allocation, but also to innovation and diffusion of new technologies. Furthermore, not enough is known about what patients want from their health care system or what health care they would choose if they were provided with objective information and, when necessary, empathic sharing by their physician of the decision-making responsibility. Until such information is obtained, along with reliable assessments of the effectiveness of available and emerging technologies, policymakers and innovators will be "flying blind"—along with doctors and patients—as they try to make health care more efficient and effective.

THE PATIENT'S PREDICAMENT: LOW BACK PAIN

All decisions, including those related to health care, are goal oriented. Common health care goals are to maintain good health and functioning, or to relieve morbidity that has decreased well-being or diminished functional capacity. Different people, however, have different life goals shaped by different circumstances, as well as different values and preferences. These in turn shape their particular health care wants and needs.

When faced with the risk of, or actual, illness, most people without professional medical training do not have the information necessary to understand their particular health care predicament or the diagnostic and treatment options available to them. They must rely on a physician or other professional for this technical information. To ensure that the decision reflects the patient's personal health care goals, he or she must understand and communicate preferences or underlying value judgments, or both, regarding the relevant health care outcomes.

Dependence on the health care professional for information and for empathic understanding of values and preferences puts a premium on trust in this relationship. Sometimes the doctor can easily and correctly infer what is best for a particular patient because the decision involves such widely shared goals that it requires little in the way of quality-of-life trade-offs; but these straightforward decisions may well be the exceptions. The following clinical example may offer some insights. Consider the predicament of a 41-year-old male physician who exercised regularly and was in excellent health until he suddenly developed low back pain. In the ensuing weeks, back pain was largely replaced by pain in the left leg extending to the ankle; there was minimal weakness of the left hamstring muscles. Bed rest for three weeks provided little relief. A magnetic resonance image disclosed a herniation of the L5-S1 intervertebral disc impinging on the left S1 nerve root.

This patient faces a choice between surgery or nonsurgical therapy. If he chooses surgery, the most likely outcome will be symptom relief, but there is a chance of a surgical complication with a serious result, even death. There is also a chance that surgery will fail and that pain will persist or worsen; if it is due to scarring in the wrong place, it may well be permanent. If the patient chooses continued nonsurgical therapy, the symptoms may disappear spontaneously, but it is more likely that he will continue to live with discomfort, at least for the next few years.

What does this patient need to know to make the right decision? What does his doctor need to know to help him with that process? First, he needs to know the probabilities of the different outcomes noted above. Where does this information come from? Often, such probabilities are derived from the relatively limited experience of the clinician, supplemented by what he learns from others and can glean from the published literature. Based on multiple interviews with scores of back surgeons and physicians, this author can attest to wide variability in the estimates that would be provided to this man.

The literature does not offer very much in the way of help. Experienced surgeons readily acknowledge an important publication bias that sometimes produces unwarranted enthusiasm for surgery among their younger colleagues. Data are available from only one randomized trial related to this condition; the trial was performed in Norway 20 years ago with a total of 126 patients, 60 of whom were randomly selected to undergo surgery (Weber, 1983). The paucity of information is surprising, considering that approximately 500,000 people face this decision and 200,000 find their way to surgery each year in the United States alone. Furthermore, the results of the Norwegian study may not apply to this particular patient. He may be quite different from those patients who were willing to be randomized, with a different clinical syndrome and comorbid factors. As a result, he may face quite different outcome probabilities.

Additional questions can be raised about the adequacy of the information base, because the clinical decision problem is more complicated than what has been portrayed thus far. There are actually many choices to be made, between new and old diagnostic tests and new and old therapies. The first surgery for herniated disc was performed at Massachusetts General Hospital some 60 years ago; a handful of cases were reported by Mixter and Barr in the *New England Journal of Medicine* in 1934, some 40 years before the only randomized trial. Consider the technologies that have come and gone, or come and stayed, since that trial: technologies to improve diagnostic acumen, such as myelograms (most recently with water-soluble contrast media), discography, computed tomography (CT) scans, and now magnetic resonance imaging, or MRI; added to these are agents or procedures for treatment, such as chymopapain, microsurgery, and even percutaneous removal of disc material. When surgeons agree on the need for surgery, they often disagree on which procedure should be chosen from the myriad approaches available involving variations of discectomy alone, or discectomy combined with laminectomy, foraminotomy, or fusion (Deyo et al., 1991). Because of these differences, and perhaps because of differences in skill, different providers produce different outcomes, which result in different outcome rates. Neither providers nor patients have access to this kind of information in the current health care economy.

Even when clinical trials are rigorously conducted, the special skills of an operator or the enthusiasm of an innovator may bias results. Ten years ago, there was considerable interest in the use of chymopapain to treat lumbar disc disease. In 1982, 108 patients were treated in seven centers in a double-blind placebo-control trial. The variation in outcomes reported from these centers was striking. In several centers, administration of a placebo resulted in an outcome equal to or better than chymopapain. In others, chymopapain was dramatically effective; in fact, in one center, 100 percent of active-agent patients were deemed successes, compared with none of the placebo patients. The overall results of the trial were positive, and their submission to the Food and Drug Administration led to approval of the compound for treating lumbar disc disease; that was followed by what one skeptical surgeon called "an unprecedented stampede with 6,000 orthopedic and neurologic surgeons lined up to take a one-day course on how the extract of papaya juice should be injected into the human back" (Fager, 1984).

Recognition of the inadequate and limited mechanisms available to maintain and enhance the professional knowledge base has led to the establishment of the Agency for Health Care Policy and Research, with its emphasis on outcomes research. The agency's main objective is a continuously improving professional knowledge base complete with outcome probabilities to aid decision making and comparative rates to stimulate examination and improvement of applications of technology.

So there are problems with the knowledge base, and clearly patients have a stake in accurate, objective information. But that is not all the patient needs; he must also determine how he feels about the alternative outcomes. Patients who face the same probabilities may make different choices because they assign different values to the same outcomes (Sackett and Torrance, 1978; Mulley, 1989).

A brief aside is warranted here to introduce a notion that is important in considering policies drawn from a bureaucratic model of resource allocation. In developing decision guidelines that include patients' preferences for different health outcomes, some number of patients might be interviewed. Previous work of this kind has demonstrated repeatedly that in doing so one would find a rather wide distribution of responses. As researchers aggregate those responses to incorporate a utility into their decision model or implicit consensus process, they might use an average value. This approach allows them to scale the health states; it also provides preferences for a hypothetical average patient. The clinician's job is not to scale health states but to discriminate among patients who have different relative preferences for the relevant outcomes.

The decision analyst might be satisfied with the probabilities and utilities—and would choose the alternative with the highest expected utility. But few people make decisions based on expected utility; instead, they exhibit varying degrees of risk aversion when health, or life itself, is at stake. Most people are averse to risk, and there is some evidence that patients are systematically more risk averse than their doctors. The variable time preferences of individuals must also be considered. The evidence that is available suggests that patients with herniated discs do just as well in the long run with or without surgery. The benefit of surgery is quicker relief from symptoms. Patients must thus weigh the value they place on early relief against a greater risk of longer-term chronic pain.

Interviews with patients who suffer from low back pain have explored the interactions of these patients with their doctors during the treatment decision-making process. These interviews indicate substantial variability in how patients and physicians deal with these difficult communication issues. Generally, patients want information. But they also want to be able to trust their doctors to help them decide what is best for them. This issue is discussed more fully later.

THE PATIENT'S PREDICAMENT: EARLY BREAST CANCER

Let us consider a second case. A 42-year-old mother of two children considered herself quite healthy until 2 weeks ago when she discovered a suspicious lump in her right breast. She has since had a mammogram, which showed a 2.5-centimeter nodule consistent with cancer. A needle biopsy confirmed the diagnosis of invasive ductal carcinoma. She has no clinical adenopathy, and her tumor is estrogen-receptor negative. Her axillary nodes were negative when examined at the time of surgery.

This woman, and about 150,000 like her each year in the United States, face two sequential decisions. Should she have a mastectomy or lumpectomy and radiation therapy as local treatment? Should she receive adjuvant therapy to reduce the chances of the tumor recurring? She too needs information. For the first decision, the probabilities are quite straightforward. The best available evidence suggests that the alternative local therapies are equivalent in terms of risk of complications and effectiveness (Fisher et al., 1985). The decision really hinges on several other factors: how the woman feels about the longer duration of lumpectomy/radiation therapy; how she feels about the risks of having a new tumor or recurrence in the preserved breast; and, most important, how she feels about keeping her breast.

For decades, this has been a controversial clinical decision. In the 1890s, William Stuart Halsted reasoned that the best chance for curing breast cancer was offered by wide excision of the breast and surrounding tissue including muscles and lymph nodes. This untested hypothesis dominated treatment for 80 years but came under increasing scrutiny in the early 1970s. Throughout the 1970s, the frequency of the Halsted operation declined steadily; the procedure was replaced by modified mastectomies that were far less disfiguring. During the 1980s, reports appeared of partial mastectomy or even simple removal of the tumor itself. These breast preservation procedures were not standardized, but when teamed with radiation therapy, they seemed to provide survival benefits equivalent to mastectomy. Some have argued that the slow diffusion of the breast preservation approaches reflects a collective indifference on the part of a largely male profession to the quality-of-life issues important to female patients. Others argue that conservatism is appropriate when the decisions are a matter of life and death. In the United States, data are unavailable on how many women would choose one option or the other. However, there is good evidence to suggest that women generally get the procedure that their surgeon prefers (Osteen et al., 1992).

The adjuvant therapy decision is equally controversial (Himel et al., 1986). Until 1988, women without evidence of tumor in their axillary lymph nodes generally were not treated with adjuvant chemotherapy. In that year, however, a clinical advisory was issued by the National Cancer Institute, based on the unpublished results of a randomized trial. When those results were published and were considered in the context of other evidence, the case for adjuvant therapy was less than compelling. Approximately 70 percent of women with early breast cancer are cured by local treatment. But it is impossible to predict which women will or will not have a recurrence; each faces a risk of recurrence of about 4 percent each year. Adjuvant therapy, the evidence suggests, will reduce that risk by approximately 30 percent, to a level of about 3 percent (Hillner and Smith, 1991). But adjuvant therapy exacts a heavy toll, conferring significant morbidity for 6 months or longer. Again, there are no data on how many women would choose adjuvant therapy if they were provided with objective information.

The communication barriers are formidable. Just one example is the distinction between the absolute and relative risk difference. Should a woman be told that adjuvant therapy will reduce her risk of recurrence by 30 percent (the relative risk difference) or that it will reduce it from an annual rate of 4 percent to 2.8 percent (the absolute risk difference)? Focusing on the risk and the relative reduction makes the benefits seem quite important. Focusing on the absolute risk difference makes the benefits seem smaller and raises a question of whether they justify the harm of chemotherapy.

One careful examination of the adjuvant therapy decision-making process at a tertiary care center (Siminoff et al., 1989) provides some insights about the very real barriers to both communication about therapeutic options and evaluation of new therapeutic regimens. In general, the women who were studied were poorly informed. They tended to substantially overestimate the benefits of adjuvant therapy as they followed the recommendations of their oncologists. Forty-eight percent of the women in the study were advised to have therapy that would be considered standard for their node status and menopausal status; 98 percent of these women followed that recommendation. Thirty percent of the women were advised to follow what were considered nonstandard recommendations, which were usually part of a treatment arm of another ongoing trial; 80 percent of these women complied with those recommendations. Twenty-two percent of the women were advised to participate in one of three ongoing trials; of these, only 46 percent agreed to do so.

Close examination of the content of the interviews led the author of this paper to speculate on the reasons for this singular exception to patients' willingness to comply with recommendations. The interviews suggested that the recommendation of the oncologist was often half-hearted or not supported by the information that was communicated. Oncologists often recommended standard or less aggressive nonstandard therapy to women with better prognoses (e.g., fewer positive nodes), and recommended more aggressive nonstandard therapy to women with worse prognoses. In essence, the oncologists often behaved as if the question being addressed by the trial had already been answered. They discussed trade-offs between present and future patients, with the edge always going to the identified former rather than the unidentified latter. Doctors were overly confident about what they knew, and patients were overly optimistic about how much they would benefit. Neither had an incentive to invest in new knowledge.

THE PROFESSIONAL MODEL: ROLE AND RESPONSIBILITIES

The two exemplary cases discussed above indicate that patients have a stake in a continuously improving base of medical knowledge that depends not only on clinical trials but also on the orderly collection of information from representative clinical practice. They also have a stake in being treated like individuals with wants and needs that may be different from those of seemingly similar people. They need objective information, or a doctor who has such information, as well as help in dealing with the subjective variables that may be as important or more important in determining the care that is best for them.

This formulation implies a set of responsibilities for patients and doctors—and for policymakers. The heaviest burden falls on the medical profession as the keeper of the ever-changing knowledge base. Clearly, it must do a better job of securing and making good use of both outcome probabilities and comparative outcome rates. The profession also has the privilege of helping people with some of their most personal decisions. It must do a better job of sharing this collective vicarious experience with those who could benefit.

What about patients? The patient's role in this model is not the passive sick role that Parsons described in 1951. Do patients want information? Are they willing to face risks and participate in decision making? A small but interesting body of literature addresses these questions (Brody, 1980; Strull et al., 1984; Ende et al., 1989). The responses can be fairly summarized as "yes" and "it depends." Patients generally want information whether or not they are prepared to bear responsibility for decisions. In fact, a number of anecdotes have been cited repeatedly to make the point that many patients do not want decision-making responsibility, particularly when the condition is serious (Inglefinger, 1980). The studies that have been conducted, however, provide conflicting evidence.

Most studies that have addressed the decision-making question have not assured patients that they will be provided with the information necessary to participate in an informed decision. When that information is provided, patients accept decision-making responsibility. For a woman facing a new diagnosis of breast cancer, it is a difficult time to bear the responsibility for making a decision; nevertheless, when 153 women with early-stage breast cancer were given a choice between breast preservation and mastectomy in Newcastle, England, none declined to decide for herself (Wilson et al., 1988). Interestingly, 65 percent of the women chose mastectomy; most cited a wish to get the treatment behind them quickly and a reluctance to face the risk of future cancer in the same breast.

Furthermore, there is emerging evidence that patient involvement in care has a positive impact on patient reports of treatment outcome and on objective measures of it (Greenfield et al., 1985, 1988; Kaplan et al., 1989). But information is not a substitute for empathy and concern—and alone, it will not establish a basis for trust. For the patient, these may be the most important attributes of a health care encounter. The most consistent finding in the voluminous patient satisfaction literature is that those characteristics of the provider and his or her organization that make care more personal are associated with higher levels of satisfaction (Cleary and McNeil, 1988). Good communication skills, empathy, and caring are the strongest predictors of patient-perceived quality of care.

What about the role of policymakers? This function legitimately comprises the need to establish constraints, including economic constraints. More information about what patients want could be valuable in this regard, empowering policymakers in a way that they have not been empowered before. Policymakers, however, also have the responsibility to provide those mechanisms and services that constitute public goods. The kind of objective information system described in this paper is a public good.

MARKET AND BUREAUCRATIC MODELS:
THE PATIENT'S STAKE

How have changes in the health care economy changed the patient's stake in that economy? As indicated earlier, the forces of policy change have been moving in two directions, both of which represent efforts to improve efficiency. The first has been toward increased competition—that is, the market model. Such policies shift the burden and responsibility for accurate information to patients.

The greatest danger of this approach is that competition may further compromise the quality of information available to patients and to the profession. Proprietary interests, competition on the basis of perceived rather than established quality, and development of unrealistic expectations before the point of sale all conspire against objective information, informed decision making, and efficient resource allocation. Policies that promote competition have sanctioned deviations from the professional model that facilitate persuasion through manipulation of values and preferences as well as selective use of information.

The problems for patients are quite different with policies drawn from the bureaucratic model—that is, what Wennberg and Barer and Evans elsewhere in this volume have called "micromanagement of care." Efforts to reduce variation and to reduce induced demand for unnecessary care characterize this approach. For patients, the danger here is not so much related to the objectivity of the information used for decision making as it is to the potential for neglecting subjective variables. Value judgments, which are necessarily aggregated in order to make policy decisions, may actually be unrepresentative of the vast majority of individuals. The resulting policies will be inefficient because some patients will receive care that they themselves would never choose to receive and others will go without care they want. This is not to say that the health care economy, in this country or in others, does not need real constraints. Management of the supply of care, in the form of decisions to invest or disinvest in the capacity of the system to provide various services to a population, justifiably depends on societal value judgments and group norms.

An additional concern about the growing tendency to manage individual care decisions is the potential for further depersonalization of care and diminishment of the complex trust relationship between doctors and patients. This relationship is often quite important to many patients as they are made vulnerable by illness, and it is of equal importance to many physicians as a source of professional gratification. Silberman addresses these themes in the next paper.

REFERENCES

Brody, D. S. 1980. The patient's role in clinical decision-making. *Annals of Internal Medicine* 93:718-722.

Cleary, P. D., and McNeil, B. J. 1988. Patient satisfaction as an indicator of quality. *Inquiry* 25:25-36.

Deyo, R., Cherkin, D., Loeser, J., Bigos, S., and Ciol, M. 1991. Lumbar spine fusion: Geographic variations, costs and consequences. *Clinical Research* 39:315A.

Ende, J., Kazis, L., Ash, A., and Moskowitz, M. A. 1989. Measuring patients' desire for autonomy: Decision making and information seeking preferences among medical patients. *Journal of General Internal Medicine* 4:23-30.

Fager, C. A. 1984. The age-old back problem. *Spine* 9:326-328.

Fisher, B., Bauer, M., Margolese, R., Poisson, R., Pilch, Y., Redmond, C., et al. 1985. Five-year results of a randomized clinical trial comparing total mastectomy with or without radiation in the treatment of breast cancer. *New England Journal of Medicine* 312:665-673.

Friedson, E. 1990. The centrality of professionalism to health care. *Jurimetrics* 30:431-445.

Greenfield, S., Kaplan, S., and Ware, J. 1985. Expanding patient involvement in care: Effects on patient outcomes. *Annals of Internal Medicine* 102:520-528.

Greenfield, S., Kaplan, S. H., Ware, J. E., Yano, E. M., and Frank, H. J. 1988. Patients' participation in medical care: Effects on blood sugar control and quality of life in diabetes. *Journal of General Medicine* 3:448.

Hillner, B. E., and Smith, T. J. 1991. Efficacy and cost-effectiveness of adjuvant chemotherapy in women with node-negative breast cancer. *New England Journal of Medicine* 324:160-168.

Himel, H. H., Liberati, A., Gelber, R. D., and Chalmers, T. C. 1986. Adjuvant chemotherapy for breast cancer. *Journal of the American Medical Association* 256:1148-1159.

Inglefinger, F. J. 1980. Arrogance. *New England Journal of Medicine* 303:1507-1511.

Kaplan, S. H., Greenfield, S., and Ware, J. 1989. Assessing the effects of physician-patient interactions on the outcomes of chronic disease. *Medical Care* 27:S110-S127.

Mixter, W. J., and Barr, J. S. 1934. Rupture of the intervertebral disc with involvement of the spinal canal. *New England Journal of Medicine* 211:210-215.

Mulley, A. G. Jr. 1989. Assessing patients' utilities: Can the ends justify the means? *Medical Care* 27:S269-S281.

Mulley, A. G. Jr. 1990. Medical decision making and practice variation. In: Andersen, T. F., and Mooney, G., eds. *The Challenges of Medical Practice Variation.* London: MacMillan.

Mulley, A. G. Jr. 1991. Finding common ground. *HMQ* 13:16-20.

Osteen, R. T., Steele, G. D., Jr., Menck, H. M., and Winchester, D. P. 1992. Regional differences in surgical management of breast cancer. *CA: The Cancer Journal for Clinicians* 42(1):39-43.

Parsons, T. 1951. *The Social System.* New York: Free Press.

Sackett, D. L., and Torrance, G. W. 1978. The utility of different health states as perceived by the general public. *Journal of Chronic Diseases* 31:697.

Siminoff, L. A., Fetting, J. H., and Abeloff, M. D. 1989. Doctor-patient communication about breast cancer adjuvant therapy. *Journal of Clinical Oncology* 7:1192-1200.

Strull, W. B., Lo, B., and Charles, G. 1984. Do patients want to participate in medical decision-making? *Journal of the American Medical Association* 252:2990-2994.

Weber, H. 1983. Lumbar disc herniation: A controlled, prospective study with ten years of observation. *Spine* 8:131-140.

Wennberg, J. E., Barnes, B. A., and Zubkoff, M. 1982. Professional uncertainty and the problem of supplier-induced demand. *Social Science Medicine* 16:811-824.

Wilson, R. G., Hart, A., and Dawes, P. J. D. K. 1988. Mastectomy or conservation: The patient's choice. *British Medical Journal* 297:1167-1170.

11

What Is It Like to Be a Patient in the 1990s?

Charles E. Silberman

To be invited to write a paper for this volume is a humbling experience for a layman. Fortunately, the subject I have been assigned—what it is like to be a patient—is one on which I can honestly claim expertise. My expertise comes from what anthropologists might call involuntary participant-observer research, conducted most recently in June of 1990, when I went into shock because of a never-before-reported toxic reaction to niacin. I conducted field research on three prior occasions as well: in November of 1985, when I underwent a laminectomy to relieve nerve compression in the spine; in January of 1988, when I had surgery to remove a malignant prostate gland; and 19 days after the prostatectomy, when I was rehospitalized with a brain stem infarct attributed to postsurgical hypercoagulability.

I recognize that personal experience can be limiting as well as illuminating. Over the past 5 years, I have read widely and deeply in the literature on medical care and health policy; I have accompanied medical school faculty on teaching rounds, observed physicians practicing in fee-for-service and health maintenance organization (HMO) settings, and in the fashion of journalists "picked the brains" of physicians, patients, administrators, policymakers, and researchers. I draw on all this in answering the question, What is it like to be a patient in the 1990s?

THE VIEW FROM THE PATIENT'S SIDE OF THE BED

In the ways that matter most, being a patient in the 1990s is exactly like being a patient in the 1980s, 1970s, or 1960s. There is a universality to the experience of illness that transcends differences in time and space, in medical technology, and in the way medical care is organized and financed. Wherever or whenever one is a patient, serious illness presents itself as an assault on one's identity and sense of self—an assault involving disorientation and loss of meaning, erosion of autonomy and control, and fear and dependency.

Sickness is a transforming experience as well, and the transformation is most evident when sickness is chronic or progressive or when it leaves us with a permanent disability. Even if "recovery" occurs, however, we do not return to our pre-sickness state; we must adjust to a new way of seeing and relating to the world. This does not mean, however, that to be a patient is to be a victim; no matter how sick or disabled, we retain the ability to choose how to respond to the situation in which we find ourselves. Hence sickness can bring gain as well as loss, for example, a more profound appreciation of spouse and children, a deeper religious faith, a clearer sense of what really matters in one's life. For the patient, in short, disease is always an existential process.

To the physician, on the other hand, disease is a pathophysiological process—under the dominant biomedical model, a process that is abstracted from the patient and his or her sufferings. In the formulation of physician Donald W. Seldin, "Human problems and human agonies are medical problems and medical illnesses only when they can be approached by the theories and techniques of biomedical science." The underlying assumption of this reductionist approach "is that all disease is physiology gone astray. Where there is truly no physiological problem, there is no disease." The extraordinary clarity and detail of the images produced by computed tomography, or CT, scans, by magnetic resonance imaging (MRI), and by other marvels of diagnostic technology reinforce this tendency to think of disease in purely organic terms (Seldin, 1981; Zucker, 1981; Reiser, 1987).

There is a world of difference, therefore, between the way most physicians think about disease and the way most patients experience it—a difference physicians often discover when they become seriously ill themselves. "I practiced medicine for fifty years before I became a patient," Edward E. Rosenbaum, former chief of rheumatology at Oregon Health Sciences University, has written. "It wasn't until then that I learned that the physician and patient are not on the same track. The view is entirely different when you are standing at the side of the bed from when you are lying in it" (Rosenbaum, 1988).

Physicians, for example, sees multiple sclerosis, or MS, as "a slowly progressive CNS [central nervous system] disease characterized by disseminated patches of demyelination in the brain and spinal cord, resulting in multiple and varied neurologic symptoms and signs, usually with remissions and exacerbations" (*Merck Manual*, 1987). That is not how MS patients experience the disease. "What I experience every day is not the demyelination in the white matter of the nervous system," philosopher Kay Toombs explains, "but . . . the ongoing and seemingly relentless diminishment of physical abilities which is surely but gradually eroding my independence. For me multiple sclerosis is the constant effort to overcome my body's resistance in order to carry out the most mundane activities, the frustration of not being able to do the simplest of things . . . and the anguished uncertainty of a perilous future" (Toombs, 1989).

I know what Dr. Toombs means. For me, stroke was not "an intra- or extracranial interruption in arterial blood flow" (*Merck Manual*, 1987). It was the infantilizing inability to stand without collapsing to my left and the consequent inability to walk; it was the unimaginable terror that what already had happened to my hospital roommates and to the other patients in the neurology service would soon happen to me—that I would lose the ability to speak intelligibly or think intelligently, or that I would be unable to feed or dress myself.

For patients, disease never is just "physiology gone astray." "What happens when my body breaks down happens not just to that body but also to my life, which is lived in that body," writes Arthur Frank, a Canadian medical sociologist who had a massive coronary followed by testicular cancer. "When the body breaks down, so does the life." Fixing the body "doesn't always put the life back together again," Frank adds, because serious illness "leaves no aspect of life untouched. . . . Your relationships, your work, your sense of who you are and who you might become, your sense of what life is and ought to be—these all change, and the change is terrifying" (Frank, 1991).

Terrifying, as I can attest, because sickness plunges us into an abyss of meaninglessness. We can describe our pain, nausea, dizziness, fatigue, malaise, or other symptoms, but we do not know what they signify; we crave explanation, all the more so because we have not completely thrown off the primordial conviction that to be sick is to be possessed by an evil spirit. We turn to our doctors to identify that spirit—to explain what is happening—as well as to make us better. There is nothing more frightening than to feel that your symptoms cannot be explained—that what is happening to you lies outside the normal course of events.

Sickness also is disorienting, for it shatters the web of assumptions on which our lives are based. We take it for granted, for example, that our arms, legs, fingers, feet, and other organs will move according to our (usually unconscious) commands. It is only when that does not happen—when we cannot stand without falling, as happened to me after my stroke, or when an arm or leg will not move as we wish—that we discover how much of our sense of self depends on those assumptions and how disoriented we become when our body turns into an enemy rather than an ally (see, e.g., Gadow, 1982; Murphy, 1987; Toombs, 1988, 1990, 1991, 1992; Mairs, 1990).

We take it for granted, too, that we control our own fate—that life is predictable and we are immortal and that we can, therefore, plan our own future. We take these assumptions for granted precisely because they are rooted in the most primitive parts of our mind. "[A]t bottom no one believes in his own death," Freud argued. "[I]n the unconscious every one of us is convinced of his immortality" (Freud, quoted in Katz, 1984, p. 217). But accident and illness force us to acknowledge our impotence and our mortality; as Steve Fishman, a young journalist who has written eloquently about his experiences following a brain hemorrhage, puts it, "Disease gives the lie to the lies we tell ourselves" (Fishman, 1988).

Losing the protection of those "lies" is isolating as well as disorienting; we feel intensely lonely despite our greater dependence on family and friends. As Flannery O'Connor, who contracted lupus at age 25, suggested, "Sickness is a place, and it's always a place where there's no company, where no one can follow" (O'Connor, quoted in Stone, 1990).

No wonder so many patients and doctors have so much difficulty communicating with one another. As John E. Ware, Jr., of the New England Medical Center's Institute for the Improvement of Medical Care and Health puts it, "Doctors and patients are like ships passing in the night" (Ware, quoted in Friedman, 1989). "In discussing my illness with physicians," Kay Toombs reports, "it has often seemed to me that we have been somehow talking at cross-purposes, discussing different things, never quite reaching one another." For the most part, Dr. Toombs adds, "this inability to communicate does not result from inattentiveness or insensitivity but from a fundamental disagreement about the nature of illness. Rather than representing a shared reality between us, illness represents two quite distinct realities, the meaning of one being significantly and qualitatively different from the meaning of the other" (Toombs, 1987).

Both realities must be attended to, as physicians often discover when they become seriously ill themselves. Neurologist Oliver Sacks had criticized medicine for its "lack of proper attention to the full needs and feelings of patients," but he was unprepared for the magnitude of his own needs after surgery to repair "a severe but uncomplicated wound to the muscles and nerves of one leg." "A physician by profession, I had never found myself a patient before, and now I was at once physician and patient," Sacks wrote. "I had imagined my injury . . . to be straightforward and routine, and I was astonished by the profundity of the effects it had: a sort of paralysis and alienation of the leg, . . . an abyss of bizarre, and even terrifying, effects. . . . What seemed, at first, to be no more than a local, peripheral breakage and breakdown now showed itself in a different, and quite terrible, light—as a breakdown of memory, of thinking, of will—*not just a lesion in my muscle but a lesion in me* [emphasis in the original]" (Sacks, 1973, 1984). The lesion in the self may be deeper and harder to heal than the lesion in the body.

THE NEW CONSUMERISM AND TECHNOLOGICAL CHANGE

Let me anticipate a question some readers may be asking themselves: Why am I telling you all this? What does the patient's experience of illness have to do with the questions addressed in the other essays in this volume? Why talk about "the perspective of the patient" in a book that explores the ways in which "the changing health care economy" may affect technological innovation?

To a patient, the answer is self-evident: if this enormous health care enterprise is about anything, it is about serving the needs of patients. And physicians, hospitals, and manufacturers of pharmaceuticals and medical devices cannot serve the needs of patients without knowing what those needs are—without understanding how patients experience and think about illness and, therefore, what patients want and expect from medical care.

What is self-evident to patients has been anything but self-evident to doctors and other providers. True, physicians, hospital administrators, and manufacturers of pharmaceuticals and medical devices have genuinely sought to meet the needs of patients. But physicians—not patients—have defined those needs.

Physicians have done so, moreover, without asking patients what they want or think they need and without otherwise taking patients' preferences and values into account. "We acknowledge that our common interest is the patient," physician Paul M. Ellwood pointed out in his 1988 Shattuck Lecture, "but we represent that interest from such divergent, even conflicting, viewpoints that everyone loses perspective. As a result, the health care system has become an organism guided by misguided choices; it is unstable, confused, and desperately in need of a central nervous system that can help it cope with the complexities of modern medicine" (Ellwood, 1988).

Guided or misguided, the choices have been made by physicians—usually without consultation with their patients. Medical practice has been based on the delegated decision-making model and the rational agency theory from which it flows. And the rational agency theory, in turn, has been based on the assumption that "doctor knows best"—in the formulation of physician/mathematician David M. Eddy, "that whatever a physician decides is, by definition, correct."

Correct by definition because a number of other assumptions have been made: that physicians know the scientifically based norms of practice; that they know the values and preferences of their patients; that physicians are disinterested and objective scientists without preferences or biases of their own; and that they therefore choose for their patients what the patients would have chosen for themselves if they had had the same knowledge. "Like Solomon," Eddy writes, "physicians could receive patients, hear their complaints, and determine the best course of action" without anybody questioning or second-guessing doctors' decisions. On the contrary, "each physician was free, trusted, and left alone to determine what was in the best interest of each patient" (Eddy, 1990).

The other providers of health care have accepted these assumptions and have operated accordingly.

- Because physicians have been their primary source of patient referrals, hospital administrators have seen physicians, not patients, as their primary customers. As a result, hospitals have been run to satisfy the needs and desires of doctors rather (or more) than the needs and desires of patients. "Hospitals vie for physician affiliations through the provision of services that physicians appreciate," Robinson and Luft (1987) explain. "These include both personal amenities such as convenient parking, office space, and clerical services and, more importantly from an economic perspective, the acquisition of state-of-the-art clinical technologies and support staffs."

- Although patients are the ultimate consumers of medications and of most medical devices, physicians generally make the purchasing decisions. Like hospitals, therefore, manufacturers of pharmaceuticals and medical devices have developed their products and built their marketing strategies around the needs and preferences of physicians rather than of patients.

The delegated decision-making model is under attack (see the later discussion, "The Revolution in Patient-Doctor Relations"); hospitals, pharmaceutical manufacturers, and manufacturers of medical devices are being forced to take account of the perspective of patients and to come to terms with their needs and preferences. This is happening in part because patients are demanding it. We live in an age of consumerism—one in which "requests" are rapidly translated into "demands," which in turn become "rights." The change is generational as well as cultural; members of the so-called baby boom generation "want far more information, involvement, control, and choice regarding the services they buy, including medical care," than do their elders (Moloney and Paul, 1991a). Patients are increasingly reluctant to accept their traditionally passive role; they are making demands and asserting rights, a process that affects the nature, as well as the rate, of technological change.

Consider the way in which patient activism is changing the allocation of federal research funds. For example, women's groups have criticized the tendency of medical researchers to ignore the health needs of women. They have pointed to the fact that large research projects such as the Multiple Risk Intervention Trial, the Health Professionals Follow-Up Study, and the Physician's Health Study have included only male patients, as well as the fact that women do not have the same access as men to critical diagnostic and therapeutic interventions such as kidney dialysis and transplantation, diagnosis of lung cancer, and catheterization for coronary bypass surgery (American Medical Association, Council on Ethical and Judicial Affairs, 1991; Cole and Wentz, 1991; Healy, 1991a).

Responding to these complaints, the National Institutes of Health (NIH) recently established an Office of Research on Women's Health to ensure "that research conducted and supported by the NIH appropriately addresses issues regarding women's health" (Healy, 1991a). As NIH director Bernadine Healy explains, "It is now time for a general awakening. Women have unique medical problems. They have greater morbidity than men and are affected by more debilitating illness" (Healy, 1991b). Hence "the NIH has mounted a multidisciplinary, multi-institute intervention study, the Women's Health Initiative, that will address the major causes of death, disability, and frailty among middle-aged and older women, including cardiovascular disease, cancer, and osteoporosis" (Healy, 1991b).

There is nothing new, of course, about lobbying for more research; the lay lobby organized in the late 1940s by Mary Lasker and Florence Mahoney helped make NIH the predominant force in biomedical research (Starr, 1982). Lobbying has become more intense, however, and lobbyists increasingly articulate the concerns of patients and their families rather than the concerns of the research community. Witness the emergence of Alzheimer's disease as a major focus of research and treatment; since formation of the Alzheimer's Disease and Related Disorders Association (ADRDA) in 1979, federal funding for research on the disease has increased 40-fold, from $4.2 million in 1979 to $80 million in 1989, despite opposition from NIH (Fox, 1989). Witness, too, the extraordinary increase in federal funding of research on the acquired immune deficiency syndrome (AIDS); by fiscal year 1990, such funding exceeded the amount allocated to research on heart disease and approached the sum allocated to cancer research (Fumento, 1990).

Patient activism has also forced significant changes in the way the Food and Drug Administration (FDA) regulates the testing and introduction of new medications. And FDA procedures, in turn, have ramifications beyond the well-being of patients or of pharmaceutical manufacturers. Because the FDA controls the entry of all chemical compounds into clinical research, the agency "inevitably controls and potentially limits the opportunity for . . . scientific progress in medicine" (Oates and Wood, 1989). Thus, recent changes in FDA procedures provide an important case study of how the "new consumerism" may affect the development and diffusion of medical technology.

The FDA is susceptible to pressure because it is expected to balance two conflicting and sometimes incompatible goals: encouraging technological innovation by making sure that effective remedies become available as quickly and as widely as possible; and protecting patients against ineffective, as well as unsafe, medications and medical devices—a mandate that tends to slow the pace of innovation (see, e.g., Kessler, 1989; Lasagna, 1989). Specifically, the federal Food, Drug, and Cosmetic Act gives the FDA power to require "substantial evidence" that a new medication (and since 1976, a new medical device) is "safe" and "effective" before it can be sold in the United States.

Lobbying is almost inevitable because of the wide discretion the FDA enjoys. As Gelijns and Thier (1990) point out, "The Food, Drug, and Cosmetic Act allows considerable latitude for subjective interpretation of the terms 'safety' and 'effectiveness' in determining the acceptable risk-benefit ratio" that a manufacturer must demonstrate before a new drug is approved. Since the 1962 amendment to the act, the FDA has attached a higher priority to protecting patients against new drugs than to making new remedies available; as Louis Lasagna puts it, "The FDA prides itself on being the most demanding regulatory agency in the world and seems remarkably unconcerned about any drug lag that might result from [its] typical snail-like pace" (Lasagna, 1989).

More is involved than pride; until recently, political pressures impelled the FDA to emphasize safety rather than speed. "It is rare for top FDA officials to be called on the congressional carpet for failing to approve a drug but common for them to have to defend having allowed a drug on the market that produced unexpected serious toxicity," Lasagna explains. "As a former FDA examiner put it, 'Any time you approve a new drug, you're wide open for attack. If it turns out to be less effective than the original data showed, they can nail you for selling out to a drug company. If it turns out to be less safe than anybody expected, some congressman or a newspaper writer will get you. So there's only one way to play it safe—turn down the application. Or at least stall for time and demand more research.'"

Time is the one thing patients with AIDS or other incurable diseases do *not* have. "When there is no alternative treatment for a life-threatening disease, a greater emphasis may need to be placed on accelerating development than on ensuring every aspect of safety and effectiveness," David A. Kessler, the physician/lawyer who now serves as FDA commissioner, pointed out in a 1989 article. The FDA began to shift its emphasis in the early 1980s in response to growing assertiveness on the part of patients with life-threatening and/or incurable diseases and as a result of ideological pressures for deregulation. By creating the category of Group C drugs, the agency allowed desperately ill cancer patients to use promising drugs that were under study but that had not yet been fully tested or approved; the FDA occasionally did the same for patients with other serious or fatal illnesses (Young et al., 1988). A precedent already had been set, therefore, when the full magnitude of the AIDS epidemic became evident.

AIDS is different from other diseases because of its virulence and epidemic proportions, and because it affects a well-organized group with considerable political skills honed in the struggle for gay rights. The result has been a quantum increase in patient activism and a sharpening of the debate over "a question that has long plagued [the FDA]: Do patients who suffer from life-threatening disorders for which there is no treatment have a right to take unproved remedies?" (Kessler, 1989; see also Hamburg and Fauci, 1989).

Under pressure from AIDS activists, who "mix antiestablishment politics with a desperate faith in the products of medical technology" (Aronowitz, 1991), the FDA began to answer in the affirmative. In 1987, for example, the agency established new "Treatment IND" (investigational new drug) application procedures to bring "promising new drugs to desperately ill patients as early in the drug's development as possible, and well before general marketing would normally provide" (Nightingale, 1987). Under the new rules, physicians were able to use investigatory drugs to treat patients with "immediately life-threatening diseases" (advanced AIDS, advanced congestive heart failure, advanced metastatic refractory cancers) or other "serious diseases" (e.g., Alzheimer's disease, advanced multiple sclerosis, progressive ankylosing spondylitis). The FDA also formalized an earlier policy permitting such patients to import unapproved drugs for their own use and expanded the policy by allowing such imports to be mailed. As David J. Rothman and Harold Edgar (1990) put it, "The agency that refused to permit the importation of laetrile to treat cancer is now on the record as saying that consumers are free to import a drug of choice if it is for their own use" (see also Halm and Gelijns, 1991).

Rothman and Edgar interpret this change as acceptance of the notion that patients should be free to make their own decisions about the use of experimental drugs based on their own assessment of benefit and risk. "It is no longer the experts who will decide, unilaterally, which risks are worth assuming," they write. "Instead, the patient, with help from physicians and other consumers, will be determining which drugs to take or not to take in the war against disease."

The change is not that far-reaching; the FDA is not relinquishing its authority, nor can it without violating its congressional mandate. The pendulum is bound to keep swinging, therefore, and patients and their advocates will continue to press the FDA to speed up the approval process and to give patients the right to decide what risks they are willing to assume.

More is changing, however, than FDA procedures; AIDS activists—and following their lead, advocates for patients with Alzheimer's disease, cancer, and other serious illnesses—have questioned the goals and methods of clinical research. Their questions in turn are forcing clinical researchers and epidemiologists to reexamine their own approach. As a group of prominent government and academic AIDS researchers acknowledged in the *New England Journal of Medicine*, "Statisticians and clinicians involved in the design and conduct of trials of new treatments for the acquired immunodeficiency syndrome (AIDS) have realized that some traditional approaches to the clinical-trials process may be unnecessarily rigid and unsuitable for this disease" (Byar et al., 1990). Specifically, "trials were relentlessly pursued as originally designed, even if data appeared outside the trial suggesting that patients would do better with a different type of management" (Merigan, 1990). The criticism is equally applicable to research on other fatal or otherwise incurable diseases.

The conduct of AIDS research has changed more rapidly because well-organized AIDS activists have forced creation of "a partnership of patients, their advocates, and clinical investigators in the AIDS Clinical Trials Group." As Thomas C. Merigan of the Stanford University Center for AIDS Research explains, "The changes stem from a shared desire that the control group receive the most up-to-date care in all clinical trials—a principle developed in cancer therapy." That in turn means that "protocols must be changed in mid-stream" to ensure that none of the patients receive inferior treatment, and that "all patients should have an equal opportunity to enter trials, even if they have disease complications or are members of a small subgroup" (Merigan, 1990).

Some now question the ethical propriety of the randomized clinical trial itself. For example, Hellman and Hellman (1991) argue that "randomized trials often place physicians in the ethically intolerable position of choosing between the good of the patient and that of society." In their view, conflict is inevitable. The practicing physician should be "primarily concerned with each patient as an individual," whereas "the clinical scientist is concerned with answering questions—i.e., determining the validity of formally constructed hypotheses." Thus, the purpose of the randomized clinical trial is "not to deliver therapy," as Anthony S. Fauci, director of the National Institute of Allergy and Infectious Diseases, acknowledges. "It's to answer a scientific question so that the drug can be available for everybody once you've established safety and efficacy." Hellman and Hellman urge physicians to shun randomized trials and adopt "other techniques of acquiring clinical information"—techniques that would enable the doctor to serve the interests of both the patient and scientific knowledge.

THE DEMAND FOR ACCOUNTABILITY

Manufacturers of pharmaceuticals and medical devices, as well as physicians and hospital administrators, will pay more attention to patient preferences for two other reasons: competitive pressures are requiring, and public and private third-party payers are demanding, that they do so. Because of escalating costs, for example, payers have begun to question the value of the medical care for which they pay. They are asking what the outcomes of medical and hospital care are and whether these are the outcomes patients want or need.

The consequences are already apparent. Physicians and hospital administrators no longer enjoy unfettered discretion in choosing the medical equipment and devices they or their patients will use; the Health Care Financing Administration (HCFA) is beginning to require evidence that a new device is cost-effective before authorizing reimbursement for Medicare patients. As a result, HCFA's coverage decisions are becoming an increasingly important factor in the development process. These coverage decisions in turn increasingly are based on more than the subjective opinions of panels of medical experts. Instead, "there is a tendency to consider the effects of devices on the quality of life of patients (including their preferences for certain outcomes)" (Gelijns, 1990).

Pharmaceutical manufacturers are facing similar pressures. To control escalating health care expenditures, private and public third-party payers now insist on more extensive evidence that a new drug or device is worth the incremental cost. Drug companies are also discovering that evidence that a drug improves the quality of patients' lives gives it a distinct competitive advantage. Hence "drug companies and manufacturers of medical devices have become consumers of quality of life and health status assessments" (Bergner, 1990).

Payers' demands for accountability are affecting doctors and hospitals even more than drug companies or manufacturers of medical devices. "Practitioners used to justify their clinical choices, if at all, only to each other, and only informally," Berwick and colleagues (1990) write. "Today, managed care systems, government agencies, utilization review departments, and payers are scrutinizing care, and with decreasing reluctance asking doctors and hospitals to explain what they do and why they do it. Doctors and hospitals used to be able to count on *someone* paying for whatever they chose to do. No longer [emphasis in original]."

The need to control costs is the primary engine of change, but competitive pressures to improve quality also play an important role. As Berwick and coworkers point out, "Quality in the modern sense is *defined* as meeting the need of customers. Who better than the customers can tell us what is needed and how we are doing [emphasis in original]?" Recognition of the importance of this definition is spreading so widely among business firms that *Business Week* has labeled the 1990s the "Decade of the Customer" (cited in Moloney and Paul, 1991a).

This is the "Decade of the Customer" for hospitals, no less than for business firms. Consider the change in hospital architecture and design. "Building hospitals with the patient in mind may not sound revolutionary, but it is revolutionizing design and architecture in American health care," a trade weekly reported in a 1988 article. "Once a puzzle of pale-green hallways, hospitals today are turning toward richer colors, pretty bedspreads, comfortable furniture, atriums, skylights, fountains, courtyards and simple floor plans. It is the natural result of a growing tendency to market medicine to the consumer" (Friedman, 1988).

The same tendency is evident in the mushroom growth of hospital marketing departments. In 1986, for example, New York's Mount Sinai Medical Center hired Natel K. Matschulat, who had created New York State's "I Love New York" advertising campaign, to fill the new position of vice president for marketing and public affairs. "Miss Matschulat acknowledged that she did not know much about hospitals, but says her experience as director of New York State's promotional campaign will help her 'apply packaged-goods techniques' in selling Mount Sinai to New York," the *New York Times* reported.

The selling has been vigorous. When market research indicated that patients' choices in hospitals are heavily influenced by their judgment of the quality of the doctors who practice in it, Matschulat created a multimillion-dollar newspaper, radio, and television advertising campaign describing medical advances for which Mount Sinai doctors have been responsible. To attract more patients to its private rooms, Mount Sinai has employed a concierge to greet patients and provide services such as catering a business meeting in a patient's room; the medical center also supplies private patients with flowers, terry cloth slippers, and reclining chairs, among other amenities.

Mount Sinai is simply following the crowd. "We used to be pretty paternalistic, but now we ask consumers what they want and we try to give it to them, whether it's shorter stay maternity care or a guarantee that they'll be seen within 15 minutes when they come to the radiology department," says Anne Doll, senior vice president for marketing of Miami Valley Hospital in Dayton, Ohio. "Physicians are still the primary gatekeeper," Lauren Barnett of the American Hospital Association explains, "but consumers make more of the choices in obstetrics, cosmetic surgery, emergency room admissions, and sports medicine" (Lewin, 1987). To attract more maternity patients, for example, New York's St. Luke's-Roosevelt Hospital Center provides free baby blankets, cute T-shirts, and candlelight dinners (shrimp cocktail and filet mignon) in bed.

Marketing gimmicks and cosmetic changes will not suffice; hospitals everywhere are discovering that they must take at least some account of their patients' preferences if they are to maintain, let alone increase, their market share. As Moloney and Paul (1991b) point out, "patients are now more actively involved in choosing their care than the traditional hospital marketing model conceived. Large and growing percentages of patients surveyed report that they are actively involved with their doctor in the choice of a hospital. Others say they chose a hospital or health plan first and then chose a doctor from among those affiliated with the facility. Many also report they have recently switched hospitals or doctors or are considering doing so."

The new competitive environment is persuading many hospitals to respond to the needs and preferences of their patients. The first step is to determine what those needs and preferences are. As part of the multimillion-dollar Picker/Commonwealth Patient-Centered Care Program, for example, Louis Harris & Associates surveyed nearly 6,500 patients recently discharged from 62 nonprofit hospitals across the country. (For a discussion of the nature of the sample, see Cleary et al., 1991.) In the telephone interview, which lasted an average of 25 minutes and included some 136 questions, patients were asked about their experiences in concrete detail. For example:

• On average, how long after you requested pain medication did you get it?

• Did someone explain *why* important tests were done in a way that you could understand, or not? Before you had tests, did a doctor or nurse explain how much pain or discomfort you would have, or not?

• Were you told what you needed to know about when and how to take your medicine(s) at home, or not? Were you told about important side effects to watch for from your medicines, or not?

• Did the doctors [nurses] sometimes talk in front of you as if you weren't there?

The specificity of the questions makes it possible for hospitals to use the responses to correct specific flaws. For example, the University of Chicago Hospitals found that one patient in four was dissatisfied with pain control, a "problem score" more than double the national average; in checking with academic medical centers with better scores, hospital officials found that Chicago had lagged behind the others in installing patient-administered analgesic units. The hospital re-surveyed its patients after expanding the number of patient-administered analgesic units and found a big increase in patient satisfaction. "I wish all problems were as easy to fix as that one," says University of Chicago Hospitals president Ralph Muller (Knox, 1991).

Although many hospitals are reluctant to be surveyed or to use the results, the use of patient surveys is bound to spread. The Picker/Commonwealth Patient-Centered Care Program is making the survey available to any hospital that wants to administer it to patients and/or family members. And the for-profit Hospital Corporation of America (HCA), a pioneer in applying "continuous quality improvement" to hospital operations, has begun surveying patients at regular 6-month intervals and is using the results to improve hospital operations (Nelson, 1991; Nelson et al., 1989, 1990).

Hospitals may not have a choice. Patients are eager for comparative information. More than 90 percent of the patients responding to the Picker/Commonwealth survey felt that "information on how patients rate their hospitals" should be made available to the public; most said that such ratings would influence their choice of where to go the next time they were hospitalized (Knox, 1991; Moloney and Paul, 1991a). And patients' desire for information is likely to be met; new assessment techniques, along with improved information-processing technology, make it relatively easy to publish patients' ratings. If hospitals do not provide the information, third-party payers will; insurance companies, employers, and government agencies can conduct their own surveys and publish the data, much as the Health Care Financing Administration has been doing for the past several years with hospital mortality rates. In 5 to 7 years, the University of Chicago Hospitals' Ralph Muller predicts, "something like Consumer Reports" will provide periodic hospital evaluations to patient/consumers (Knox, 1991).

Hospitals also are beginning to use patients' assessments of their own condition to supplement traditional clinical measures. In the opinion of Jerome Grossman, president of the New England Medical Center, asking patients how they feel and function and using their answers to monitor the quality of care "represents the missing link" in the effort to figure out what constitutes value in medical care (Friedman, 1989). Indeed, Grossman and his colleagues believe that hospitals must do more than ask patients about their condition; patients' answers must be incorporated into clinical records and used to improve the quality of care. This is no easy matter. "We know how to collect data on patients' functional status and well-being for research purposes," says Allyson Ross Davies, director of the New England Medical Center's Department of Quality Assessment. "But if clinicians are to use the information, we have to collect the data more economically and in real time, and we have to learn how to use the data to improve clinical practice."[1] To do so, Grossman brought Alvin Tarlov, John E. Ware, Jr., Sheldon Greenfield, and Sherrie Kaplan, as well as Davies, to the New

---

[1]Interview with Allyson Ross Davies, Ph.D., Boston, December 3, 1990. I am relying also on conversations that day with Alvin Tarlov, M.D., Sheldon Greenfield, M.D., and Sherrie Kaplan, Ph.D., and a telephone conversation with Jerome Grossman, M.D., on November 19, 1990.

England Medical Center's Health Institute. The significance of patient assessments will be discussed more fully below.

THE REVOLUTION IN PATIENT-DOCTOR RELATIONS

The demand for accountability is transforming patient-doctor relations. Patients are not just asking questions; they are demanding an active role in decisions about their own care. This shift from delegated to shared decision making amounts to a Copernican revolution—one that is forcing physicians and hospitals to organize medical care around the perspective of the patient as well as of the physician.

A change of sorts began in the 1950s when the courts established the doctrine of "informed consent." In fact, informed consent has had little impact on patient-doctor relations; if anything, it has reinforced the paternalism and delegation of authority inherent in the old model (President's Commission for the Study of Ethical Problems in Medicine and Biomedical Research, 1982; Katz, 1984; Green, 1988). As psychiatrist/lawyer Jay Katz (1984) points out, most patients are informed only about the risks and benefits of the treatment their doctor has recommended or has already chosen for them; patients rarely are informed about the risks and benefits of alternative treatments, including the alternative of doing nothing; and patients almost never are told "about the certainties and uncertainties inherent in most treatment options."

> Most importantly, conversations with patients are not conducted in the spirit of inviting patients to share with their physicians the burdens of decision. Without such a commitment, dialogue is reduced to a monologue. Thus, what passes today for disclosure and consent in physician-patient interaction is largely an unwitting attempt by physicians to shape the disclosure process so that patients will comply with their recommendations (Katz, 1984, p. 26).

In short, informed consent has reinforced the tendency for physicians to talk *at* their patients rather than *with* them. Indeed, patients usually do not see the "informed consent" form for a hospitalization, invasive test, and/or surgical procedure until *after* they have been admitted to the hospital, which is to say, after the crucial decisions have been made. It is not surprising, therefore, that a majority (55 percent) of physicians and an overwhelming majority (79 percent) of patients think the purpose of informed consent is to protect doctors from malpractice suits (Green, 1988).

The changes now underway go far beyond the cosmetic adjustments required by informed consent; patient-doctor relations are being revolutionized by pressures from within the profession, as well as from without (see the preceding papers by Wennberg and Mulley). The findings of researchers such as Wennberg, Eddy, Ware, Greenfield, and Brook and of clinicians such as George L. Engel and Alvan R. Feinstein have destroyed the intellectual foundations on which the delegated decision-making model rests. In particular, Wennberg and Eddy have shown that physicians frequently do not know the scientifically correct way to practice medicine—not because of personal ignorance or indifference, but because *nobody* knows; medical science has enjoyed spectacular success in developing new treatments but has largely ignored the mundane task of evaluating their results.

The paucity of information about outcomes imparts a random component to medical decisions. What illness a patient is diagnosed as having, for example, depends on who is making the diagnosis and when—witness the magnitude of inter- and intra-observer variation in the interpretation of supposedly "objective" diagnostic tests. As Eddy points out, physicians looking at the same x-ray, cardiogram, angiogram, pap smear, pathology specimen, laboratory finding, or other test result disagree with one another—or with their own prior interpretation—anywhere from 10 to 50 percent of the time. Comparable variations have been found in the way doctors interpret patient histories and physical examination findings and in the treatments physicians and surgeons recommend when shown the same clinical records (Eddy, 1984, 1990; Eddy and Billings, 1988).

How a patient is treated for a given illness also depends on where that patient lives; for the patient, geography—not anatomy—is destiny. Witness the large variations Wennberg has found in the frequency with which patients are hospitalized and/or operated on for the same illness in different communities—even communities, such as Boston and New Haven, in which the overwhelming majority of physicians are affiliated with a major teaching hospital. "If the clinicians in these academic strongholds do not know the correct way of practicing medicine," Wennberg asks, "who else could know?"

The other assumptions on which the delegated decision-making model rests are equally flawed. Specifically, physicians do not know the values and preferences of their patients; nor are physicians disinterested and objective scientists without preferences or biases of their own (see the discussion of this issue below). There is no reason to assume, therefore, that physicians choose for their patients what the patients would choose for themselves. On the contrary, Wennberg, Mulley, and their colleagues have shown that when patients with benign prostatic hypertrophy are given information about the outcomes of alternative treatments and are involved in the decisions about their own care, they make strikingly different choices for themselves than their physicians make for them. In particular, patients choose surgery far less often and "watchful waiting" far more often than do their doctors.

The disjuncture between patient preferences and physician behavior is not limited to benign prostatic hypertrophy; it is evident in the care of patients with chronic diseases—the patients for whom the bulk of medical expenditures are now incurred (Stewart et al., 1989). Because they define disease in purely pathophysiological terms (see above), physicians measure success through changes in intermediate outcomes, such as blood pressure, blood sugar levels, or patency of blood vessels.

Such measures are incomplete at best and may tell the doctor little about how the patient feels or functions; in conditions such as ulcers, angina, arrhythmias, diabetes, spinal stenosis, and disk herniation, among others, there is little correlation between the severity of the organic disorder and the amount of pain or other symptoms patients experience. Indeed, biomedical data explain only 10 to 25 percent of the variance in patients' functional status or well-being (see, e.g., Fowler et al., 1988; Stewart et al., 1989; Mulley, 1990; Ware, 1990). By concentrating on intermediate outcomes, physicians "may all too easily spend years writing 'doing well' in the notes of a patient who has become progressively more crippled before their eyes" (Smith, 1983).

That is not how patients define "doing well." Most of the time, patients see the primary goal of medical care as improvement in the quality of their lives—preserving or restoring their sense of well-being and their ability to function physically (e.g., to walk a certain distance, climb stairs, dress and feed themselves) and socially (e.g., to perform their usual activities on the job, at home, or with other family and friends). "Improvement in quality of life is not only an important outcome of medical care," John P. Bunker argues, "it is the only intended outcome of most of what we do in medicine" (Bunker, 1990; see also Ware, 1990).

Physicians cannot maintain or improve the functional status of their patients unless they know which patients have what kinds of limitations. Much of the time, physicians do not know. "Health care providers collect data about functioning for virtually every body organ," John E. Ware, Jr., points out, "but none of these measures tell about the function of the entire individual." As a result, "many, if not most, clinicians do not know the functional status and well-being of their patients" (Ware, 1989; see also Connelly et al., 1989; Hall et al., 1989; Calkins et al., 1991). In a recent study, for example, both patients and their physicians were asked to describe how much difficulty the patient experienced in performing 12 specific physical and social activities. The results were striking: overall, the physicians—one group from UCLA Medical School, a second from Beth Israel Hospital in Boston—underestimated or failed to recognize 66 percent of their patients' disabilities (Calkins et al., 1991). Physicians are no better at detecting and treating depression, which seriously impairs patients' ability to function as well as their overall sense of well-being; the Medical Outcomes Study directed by Ware, Tarlov, and Greenfield found that primary care physicians detect depression in only one depressed patient in two (Wells et al., 1989a,b)

This "lack of proper attention to the full needs and feelings of patients" is due not to insensitivity or lack of concern on the part of physicians, but to what Alvan R. Feinstein calls "scientific policy," that is, the prevailing mind-set about the kind of information physicians should seek and study. By and large, physicians are taught that what cannot be readily quantified is unimportant; information about the inner thoughts and feelings of patients is considered "soft" or "subjective"—less worthy of scientific attention than "hard" or "objective" data such as the images, numbers, and tracings produced by diagnostic testing equipment. This invidious distinction between "hard" and "soft" data has produced "a deliberate reduction of the human information used in clinical science." In ignoring "soft" data, Feinstein notes, physicians ignore "all the distinctively human reactions—love, hate, joy, sorrow, distress, gratification—that differentiate people from animals or molecules" (Feinstein, 1987).

The result is that medicine focuses on outcomes of interest to physicians, rather than to patients. As Feinstein (1983) puts it,

> We appraise the palliative treatment of patients with cancer by measuring survival time, tumor size, and other paraclinical indexes. We do not regularly measure whether the patient is comfortable or miserable, functional or bed-ridden, vegetating or vibrant. We compare medical and surgical treatment for coronary heart disease by measuring survival time, patency of vessels, electrocardiographic changes, and treadmill exercise tests. We do not regularly perform scientifically credible measurements of whether the angina pectoris is still severe, whether the patient was truly made able to return to work, and whether the quality of life has otherwise improved for the patient and his family.

This happens, to repeat, not because of ignorance or indifference but because biomedical science axiomatically excludes the human domain. "In order to know the truth of the pathological fact," the historian Michel Foucault observes, "the doctor must abstract the patient" (Foucault, 1975).

The biomedical model abstracts the physician as well. In accordance with medicine's nineteenth-century conception of science, the physician is assumed to be an objective, disinterested, and thoroughly neutral observer, and the phenomenon being studied is assumed to be independent of, and unaffected by, the observer. In conducting clinical research, for example, researchers control for patient characteristics but usually ignore differences among physicians; the practice reinforces "the conviction that the physician has no therapeutic effect as a person, but is simply a conduit of pills or procedures." "Holding all physicians as equal in a trial," Spiro (1986) points out, implies "that the physician himself does not matter."

These assumptions have been shattered by the development of twentieth-century science, especially post-Newtonian physics and evolutionary biology, which has shown that the mere presence of an observer alters the phenomenon being observed (see Odegaard, 1986; Engel, 1988; Bursztajn et al., 1990). "What we observe is not nature itself," Heisenberg explained, "but the interplay between nature and ourselves. . ." (Heisenberg, 1958). Since there is no "objective" reality independent of the observer, there can be no invidious distinction between "objective" and "subjective" knowledge; nor can physicians be mere conduits through which information and treatments pass.

On the contrary, there is a subjective component to objective knowledge: physicians' biases and values affect what they observe as well as what they recommend, and the nature of the physician's relationship with the patient affects the patient's health. Equally important, there is an objective component to what we call subjective knowledge: values and feelings can be studied and measured, although doing so requires different instruments and approaches. The hallmark of hard data, after all, is consistency, that is, whether the data can be repeated by the same observer and reproduced by another. "If repeated observations by the same or different observers yield the same results," physician Richard A. Deyo points out, "the findings have the basic ingredients of 'hardness.' By this criterion, state-of-the-art questionnaires for measuring the quality of life are as hard as many common laboratory measures" (Deyo, 1991b).

It would be hard to overstate the significance of Deyo's point. Physicians now have at their disposal a number of easily used, as well as valid and reliable, instruments for assessing patients' symptoms, functional status, and sense of well being—instruments such as the SF-36 Health Status Questionnaire developed by John E. Ware, Jr., and colleagues, the Dartmouth Coop Charts, the Duke Health Profile, the Sickness Impact Profile developed by Marilyn Bergner and colleagues, and the Quality of Well-Being Scale (see Lohr, 1992; Stewart and Ware, 1992 forthcoming). The availability of these measures destroys any lingering justification for medicine's preoccupation with purely biomedical goals and measures.

Clearly, substituting patient-doctor collaboration for the old delegated decision-making model does not mean abandoning "science" for "art." It means broadening the conception of the nature of science to include the knowledge and skills usually lumped together under the rubric "art of care." "The fundamental distinction . . . is not between 'science' and 'art,'" George Engel argues, "but between thinking and proceeding scientifically and not so thinking and proceeding" (Engel, 1988; see also Bursztajn et al., 1990).

Medical questions can be approached scientifically only if medicine follows the standards of twentieth-century science and develops a more inclusive concept of clinical practice—what George Engel calls the biopsychosocial model, Ian R. McWhinney "a patient-centered clinical method," and others simply "the new paradigm" (see, e.g., Engel, 1977, 1981, 1988; McWhinney, 1988; Bursztajn et al., 1990). That in turn means recognizing that medical practice must be a joint undertaking of physician and patient (or physician and patient's surrogate).

Indeed, collaboration between patient and physician is both a scientific and ethical imperative. It is an ethical imperative, as Wennberg, Mulley, Eddy, and others point out, because most medical procedures have multiple and contradictory, as well as uncertain, outcomes and because patients differ widely in their attitudes toward risk and uncertainty and in the values they attach to various outcomes. What we have called medical judgments frequently are not that at all; they are value judgments—judgments to which physicians have much to contribute but which they are not equipped to make on their own.

Collaboration is a scientific imperative as well, because medicine involves the study and treatment of one person by another (Engel, 1988). Thus, collaboration between doctor and patient should not be limited to the choice of treatments; it should start when the patient first seeks medical help and should continue throughout the clinical encounter. Collaboration is essential, to begin with, to determine why the patient is seeking help. In primary care medicine, in particular, patient-doctor encounters usually are initiated by the patient, for reasons that are not always apparent. Without knowing why the patient has come—and patients are not always aware of the real reason themselves—the physician may identify and treat the wrong problem.

The risk is increased by the staccato, closed-ended style most physicians use in questioning their patients. In analyzing doctor-patient interactions, Beckman and Frankel (1984) found that, on average, physicians interrupted patients 18 seconds after the patient began to speak; patients were able to complete their opening statements in only 23 percent of the visits. One consequence of these interruptions is the familiar situation in which, just as the physician thinks the office visit is over, the patient asks, "Oh, by the way, Doctor, I've been having this heavy feeling in my chest. Do you think that might be important?" Most of the time patients are not being perverse; they had not been able to get the question out when the doctor was taking their history, or the doctor may not have put them at sufficient ease to enable them to ask a painful or embarrassing question.

The only way patients can tell physicians why they are seeking medical help is through dialogue. And productive dialogue cannot occur unless the physician first establishes a relationship with the patient. Thus, "the physician has no alternative but to behave in a humane and empathic manner . . . if the patient is to be enabled to report clearly and fully," Engel writes. "Only then can the physician proceed scientifically; to be humane and empathic is not merely a prescription for compassion . . . it is a prerequisite for scientific work in the clinical realm" (Engel, 1988).

We pay a heavy economic, as well as human, price for the lack of dialogue and the paucity of collaborative relations between doctors and patients. Specifically, devaluation of information from patients contributes significantly to missed diagnoses; to inappropriate and excessive use of diagnostic tests, medications, and invasive treatments; and to underuse of a significant low-tech "technology," the patient-doctor relationship.

In a highly suggestive study, for example, Everitt and colleagues (1990) asked a random sample of primary care physicians how they would treat a 77-year-old patient complaining of insomnia—a patient whom they were seeing for the first time. After the physicians were given a brief history, they were asked what additional information they needed in order to choose a treatment. Fewer than half the doctors asked for any information about the patient's sleeping pattern; had they done so, they would have learned that the patient slept seven hours a night. He had "insomnia" because he went to bed each night at 9 p.m. and could not get back to sleep when he awakened at 4 a.m. (The patient also drank two cups of regular coffee at dinner; but fewer than one physician in four asked about his caffeine consumption.)

In short, rudimentary interviewing of the patient would have suggested that the "insomnia" could be addressed without medication; yet only 15 percent of the physicians recommended cutting down on caffeine, going to sleep at a later hour, or some other change in life style. Nearly two-thirds of the physicians recommended a hypnotic or psychoactive drug such as triazolam, flurazepam, temazepam, or amitriptyline—in a 77-year-old patient they had never seen before.

In a more recent study, the same researchers (Avorn et al., 1991) found a similar pattern in the treatment of an elderly patient with abdominal pain. The physicians prescribed histamine antagonists for someone who smoked 2 packs of cigarettes and consumed 8 aspirin and 5 cups of caffeine a day.

The need for a collaborative relationship between doctors and patients is strikingly evident in the care of patients with chronic diseases. With the explosion in outcomes research, there is increasing documentation of the failures of treatments based on exclusively biomedical considerations. For example:

> The history of medical care for low back pain—one of the most common causes of morbidity and absenteeism in the United States—involves serial fashions in diagnosis and therapy. Earlier in this century, sacroiliac joint disease was thought to account for many cases of back pain, and this led to many fusions of the sacroiliac joint. Coccydynia was a popular diagnosis that led to a wave of coccygectomies, a procedure now almost completely abandoned. The use of chymopapain injections for herniated lumbar intervertebral disks enjoyed explosive growth in the early 1980s, but has declined greatly. Recent clinical trials have challenged the efficacy of many popular treatments, including lengthy bed rest, traction, and transcutaneous

electrical nerve stimulation. Each of these fashions arose from a seductive pathoanatomical theory, leading to the popularity of a diagnosis that justified the corresponding treatment. Such fads are not innocuous; they may lead to unnecessary morbidity and costs, as well as to embarrassment for professionals" (Deyo, 1991a; see also the preceding paper by Mulley).

Deyo's observations were made in an editorial commenting on a study showing the worthlessness of the most recent fad, corticosteroid injections into the facet joints (Carette et al., 1991).

One reason purely biomedical approaches often fail is that chronic illnesses involve what Greenfield and colleagues (1988) call "discretionary dysfunctioning." As already noted, the same pathophysiology is associated with widely different effects in different patients; in a sense, patients exercise discretion "in determining the extent to which the illness will compromise functioning" or affect their overall sense of well-being. Some of this discretionary dysfunctioning depends on the patient's personality and temperament and the support he or she receives from family and friends.

Much of it depends on factors physicians can influence, such as whether patients follow the prescribed treatment regimen. Physicians call this "compliance," a locution that places the blame for "noncompliance" solely on patients. But patients are not likely to carry out a complicated regimen unless their physicians persuade them of its importance. A lot of persuasion may be necessary if the medications have disagreeable side effects or if the patient must change deeply ingrained habits, lifestyles, or values. Patients cannot "comply" with a regimen, moreover, if they do not understand it—if they do not know, for example, what medications they should take, when they should take them (before, during, or after meals?), or whether they should stop the medication if they feel better or finish the bottle. If the latter, should the prescription be refilled? Clearly, the skill with which physicians relate to patients and communicate with them affects both their willingness and their ability to "comply."

How physicians relate to patients affects more than "compliance." In a series of controlled experiments with patients with diabetes, hypertension, and ulcers, Kaplan and colleagues (1989) have shown that when patients are taught to play an active role in the patient-doctor relationship, their health improves—as measured, for example, by hemoglobin $A1_c$ and diastolic blood pressure—as well as by improvements in functional status. "We can thus assert with some confidence," Kaplan and coworkers (1989) write, "that the effects we observed represent a real impact on patients' health—that patients 'aren't just saying' that their health is improved."

There should be nothing surprising about this finding; the pervasive placebo effect demonstrates the therapeutic power of the patient-doctor relationship (Brody, 1980, 1982; also Spiro, 1986). Curiously, researchers consistently ignore the benefit of the placebo and focus on the difference between the placebo effect and the supposedly active medication or treatment. Yet when so many double-blind controlled clinical trials show almost as much healing from the placebo as from the drug or procedure being tested, it is hard to escape the conclusion that the healing comes from the placebo as well as—or more than—from the drug (Spiro, 1986).

TECHNOLOGICAL INNOVATION AND PATIENT CARE

To recapitulate, American medicine is undergoing a change as far-reaching as that ushered in by the introduction of antibiotics a half century ago. This change amounts to a Copernican revolution—one that is returning the patient to the center of the medical universe.

In choosing treatments, as Wennberg and Mulley have shown, collaboration between doctor and patient is an ethical necessity. Much if not most of the time, there is no "right" or "wrong" decision about how to treat a particular condition; the right choice of treatment depends on the preferences and values of the patient in question (see Mulley, in this volume).

Replacing the delegated decision-making model with a shared decision-making model is a necessary but insufficient change. Medical practice must involve a shared clinical encounter. Collaboration between patient and doctor should begin when the patient first seeks help and continue throughout the medical encounter. Collaboration is essential for several reasons.

First, the patient is a crucial source of information for diagnosis. Second, patients are equally important sources of information on the effects of treatment, such as reduction in pain or other symptoms or improvement in functional status and well-being. The existence of valid, reliable measures for assessing patients' functional status and sense of well-being makes it scientifically, as well as ethically, intolerable for physicians to fail to be as concerned with their patients' attitudes, feelings, preferences, and values as they are with their physiological status.

This shift from disease-centered to patient-centered medicine is bound to change some of the criteria governing the development, adoption, and diffusion of new technology. As I have shown earlier, patient activism has already altered the processes by which FDA approves new drugs and HCFA decides whether to authorize reimbursement for new devices; the same pressures are forcing hospitals to pay attention to the needs and preferences of patients, rather than of physicians. There will be an equally large impact on the nature of the technologies that doctors use. One can already see a growing emphasis on technologies directed at the outcomes of particular interest to patients, such as reduction of pain or speedier recovery.

Consider the unprecedented speed with which laparoscopic cholecystectomy has been adopted; in a mere 12 to 18 months, the procedure went "from being unavailable in most communities to being a commonly used technique . . . despite very limited published data to substantiate that the laparoscopic approach is superior to the traditional procedure" (Wolfe et al., 1991). In a growing number of communities, in fact, it already has become the procedure of choice.

The rapid diffusion of this technique is a response, in part, to payers' demands for less costly alternatives to expensive procedures. For the most part, however, diffusion has been driven by patient demand; the reported advantages of the technique "include diminished postoperative pain, . . . more rapid recovery and return to full activity, and a superior cosmetic result" as well as "shorter hospitalization and associated cost" (Wolfe et al., 1991; see also the Southern Surgeons Club, 1991). Patient demand for the laparoscopic approach was so strong that plans for a prospective randomized trial at the University of California, Davis, had to be abandoned; patients were unwilling to chance being assigned to the control group (Wolfe et al., 1991). (Laparoscopic technology is now being applied to other kinds of abdominal surgery.)

Patients want more than reduction in pain and other symptoms; they want more control over their own condition and treatment, as well. Hospitals' growing use of self-administered analgesic units represents one kind of technological response to these desires; giving patients more control over the management of their own pain seems to lead to less, rather than more, use of analgesic medication.

Pharmaceutical manufacturers, meanwhile, are avidly searching for alternatives to injection for administering insulin, hormones, and other protein-based medications. Self-injection is awkward and inconvenient, and many patients with diabetes dislike having to inject themselves two or three times a day because it symbolizes their dependence and lack of control. Hence manufacturers have stepped up their efforts to develop implantable pumps, patches, and methods for spraying the medication into the nostrils or lungs (Thompson, 1990).

The interactive videodisc technology that Wennberg, Mulley, and colleagues are developing to inform patients with breast cancer, back pain, benign prostatic hypertrophy, and other conditions about treatment outcomes and to assist them in making decisions about their own care represents still another response to the rise of patient-centered medicine. Patients *need* help in making the change; the delegated decision-making model is so deeply ingrained that patients find it hard to relate to their physicians as equals and to play an active role in decisions about their own care.

Awe of the doctor is instilled in us in childhood, when we see our parents defer to the doctor and carry out his or her orders. "In the child's mind, the authority and mysterious power of the doctor supersede the authority of the parents," Thomas A. Preston of the University of Washington Medical School has written. "The physician is the only one who is allowed to violate the rules and taboos of the home, entering the bedroom and physically handling the child's body." By the time we are grown, we have "learned to accept the power of the doctor to set rules, make pronouncements, and give orders, and [we have] long since come to believe in the doctor's ability to cure" (Preston, 1986).

Even when we are well, therefore, it is hard for lay people to relate to doctors as equals; and as I have shown above, illness makes us feel vulnerable and dependent, destroying our sense of control over our lives and our bodies. Our dependency is exacerbated by our need for the doctor not only to cure us but, equally important, to help us make sense of what is happening—hence the need for reeducation if patients are to learn to relate to physicians in an egalitarian but nonconfrontational way. The interactive video technology Wennberg, Mulley, and colleagues are using is an enormously promising approach.[2]

Physicians need as much help as patients. Authoritarianism is deeply ingrained in medical education and practice and is powerfully reinforced by the dependency doctors often see in their patients. "Ever since the 1960s, we've been told that the patient must be the colleague of his doctor and that the decision making must be shared equally by them," says Richard Selzer. "Intellectually and philosophically I certainly do agree."

> Unfortunately, it doesn't quite work out that way. When I try to call the patient in on a consultation and say, "Which alternative would you prefer?" *invariably* the patient says, "What do you mean, which alternative? I want you to tell me what to do. You're the doctor." The only unspoken word is daddy; tell me what to do, daddy. When a person is desperately ill or frightened, there is a certain kind of regression that makes you want to place yourself in someone's loving care. It is the responsibility of the doctor to have the courage to make decisions for the patient, in as kind and wise a way as he can. To be a father or mother and comfort [emphasis in the original] (Selzer, quoted in Katz, 1984, p. 126).

Selzer's reaction is understandable, but he has misinterpreted his patients' needs. Frequently, a patient "will do his best to push you into the place of parental authority, and he will make use of you as a parental authority to the utmost," Anna Freud told Case Western Reserve Medical School students in a 1964 lecture. "You must understand that."

---

[2]Greenfield, Kaplan, and Ware have used a different approach in their controlled experiments studying the impact of patient activism on health (see above). In 20-minute sessions immediately preceding their visits to their doctors, patients were given information about their medical record and the treatment alternatives from which their physician would choose. Patients also received "coaching in behavioral strategies for increasing their participation in care during the office visit," including "techniques for improving question-asking and negotiating skills and ways of defusing hostility or intimidation on the part of the physician" (Kaplan et al., 1989; Greenfield et al., 1988).

On the other hand, *you must not be tempted to treat him as a child*. You must be tolerant towards him as you would be towards a child and as respectful as you would be towards a fellow adult because he has only gone back to childhood as far as he's ill. *He also has another part of his personality which has remained intact, and that part of him will resent it deeply, if you make too much use of your authority* [emphasis added]" (Anna Freud, quoted in Katz, 1984, p. 146).

It will not be easy for physicians to learn to treat patients as adults rather than as children. The technology that Wennberg and Mulley are using to educate patients could be used to reeducate physicians, as well. Other technologies may also come into play; as part of his ongoing research on the therapeutic impact of patient-doctor relations, Sheldon Greenfield made a 20-minute film (using conventional VHS technology) to teach physicians how to present treatment alternatives to patients, how to negotiate with patients, how to get passive patients involved in their own care, and so on.[3]

Patient-centered medicine will affect the development and diffusion of technology in other ways. In particular, a more patient-centered approach to medicine is likely to result in more discriminating use of technology. Until now, clinical practice has often been driven by technology, which imposed a logic of its own. Witness the so-called "cascade effect" in which one perhaps unnecessary diagnostic test leads to another, which leads to another, and so on. Here is a recent description of how the cascade effect works in cardiology.

> Instead of delving more carefully into the history when a patient presents with unusual chest pain, someone may order an exercise test that shows suspicious changes, leading to an isotope study with suggestive defects in a shadowy image, followed by arteriograms that, predictably, in most cases show some coronary disease, and so on down the cascade, sometimes with disastrous complications that no one wanted or anticipated (James, 1988; see also Mold and Stein, 1986).

All this because of failure to take a careful history.

The more tests that are done, of course, the higher the probability that the patient will be found to have some abnormality. And when an abnormality is found, the assumption that disease is pathophysiological creates a bias in favor of intervention: "Once a lesion is found there is an irresistible temptation to remove it or fix it." Hence the recurrent cycle of surgical remedies, such as gastric freezing for duodenal ulcers, ligation of the internal mammary arteries for angina, or intragastric balloons for obesity, that are discovered, tried, and then proven worthless at best and harmful at worst.

---

[3]Conversation with Sheldon Greenfield, December 3, 1990.

The tendency to substitute diagnostic tests and surgical procedures for information from, and therapeutic relationships with, patients has been exacerbated by the way in which physicians have been reimbursed. By paying doctors far higher fees for tests and procedures than for the same time and effort spent talking to patients, the insurance reimbursement system has given doctors powerful financial incentives to maximize their use of technology and avoid collaborative relationships with patients. The payment system "so favors the biotechnical aspects of care," Moloney and Paul (1991b) write, "that the implicit message to professionals is 'talk to patients on your own time.'" The income differentials resulting from the discrepancies in fees have also channeled young physicians away from the primary care disciplines of pediatrics, internal medicine, and family practice and toward procedure-oriented specialties (Physician Payment Review Commission, 1990).

The incentives are changing now as a result of the reform of the Medicare physician payment system that began in the fall of 1991. The change was proposed by the Physician Payment Review Commission, or PPRC, and mandated by Congress in 1989; although the reform is to be phased in over 5 years, the largest part of the change will be completed by the end of fiscal 1992 (Physician Payment Review Commission, 1991).

Under the new system, Medicare payments to physicians will be determined by the resources needed to provide the service in question. These resources include the physician's time, physical effort, and skill; the mental effort and judgment required; the stress that is involved; and the associated costs of that kind of practice. When implementation of the system is complete, fees for primary care services will have risen by 30 percent or more, and there will be comparable reductions in payments for major diagnostic and surgical procedures. (To discourage physicians from performing more procedures to compensate for lower fees, the legislation mandates the establishment of annual "volume performance standards"; if physicians increase volume more rapidly than the standard allows for that year, their fees would be reduced accordingly in the following year.) It is too soon to know whether insurance companies and employers will apply the concept to the private sector, but such an expansion is likely (Ginsburg and Lee, 1991).

Whether limited to Medicare or not, physician payment reform is bound to affect decisions about the use of medical technology. It will do this by creating a level playing field—one in which financial incentives neither encourage nor discourage the use of technology. But physician payment reform *will* encourage the development of a more collaborative patient-doctor relationship by rewarding doctors equally for patient-oriented and procedure-oriented activities. It may also reverse the long-term movement of physicians away from primary care and into procedure-oriented specialties.

The need is clear; how rapidly medicine adopts a more patient-centered approach will depend in good measure on the strength of the countervailing forces. As Wennberg and Mulley point out in their papers in this volume, the managed care approach to cost control implies different roles and responsibilities for the actors in the health care drama—doctors, patients, and policymakers. *How* different these roles can be was dramatized in late November 1991 when Thomas O. Pyle, the longtime chief executive of the Harvard Community Health Plan, was forced to resign by staff physicians angry over his plan to link their compensation with the number of patient visits they handled. The change would have created pressure on physicians to limit the time they spent with each patient. "Mr. Pyle's resignation underscores tensions that have developed at many health care organizations as competition for corporate and individual customers has intensified," the *Wall Street Journal* reported. "In August, top executives at Bay State Health Care, another large Boston-area HMO, resigned after a similar dispute concerning physician compensation" (Stipp, 1991). True, many HMOs try to increase physician "productivity" by limiting the time physicians can spend per patient visit. But as Robert Blendon of the Harvard School of Public Health comments, the Harvard Community Health Plan "is supposed to be a special place for special people" (Stipp, 1991).

As Samuel Goldwyn is said to have remarked, predictions are always dangerous—especially about the future. Let me run the risk: the forces underlying the shift toward a more collaborative patient-doctor relationship seem to me to be too powerful to be offset by managed care, which moves decision making away from the patient and his or her physician and toward some anonymous bureaucrat.

In the rest of the economy, after all, the trend is toward more accountability to the customer. "About two decades ago, J. D. Power changed the nature of the automotive marketplace and influenced the future design of cars as well," Moloney and Paul (1991b) point out. "He did so by making consumer ratings of various aspects of new model automobiles widely available to the public."

> Industry officials warned that this practice would lead to wasteful changes in automotive design, such as larger tail fins and more metallic paint. In fact, consumers proved industry experts wrong, choosing instead cars needing fewer repairs and offering better safety features. Patients are now eager to know how other patients rate their care. They say they would use their neighbors' ratings as a key factor in deciding where to seek care in the future. Can the day be far ahead when employers, insurers, or citizens groups sponsor surveys of patient perceptions of care received under competing medical plans, at competing hospitals or group practices, and make those reports available to patients and their insurance sponsors?

Or the day when patients and physicians collaborate and medical care is directed toward the outcomes patients want and need.

REFERENCES

American Medical Association, Council on Ethical and Judicial Affairs. 1991. Gender disparities in clinical decision making. *Journal of the American Medical Association* 266:559-562.

Aronowitz, R. A. 1991. Review of Rothman, D. J. *Strangers at the Bedside: A History of How Law and Bioethics Transformed Medical Decision Making. Journal of General Internal Medicine* 6:593-594.

Avorn, J. L. 1986. Medicine: The life and death of Oliver Shay. In A. Pifer, and L. Bronte, eds. *Our Aging Society.* New York: W. W. Norton & Company.

Avorn, J., Everitt, D. E., and Baker, M. W. 1991. The neglected medical history and therapeutic choices for abdominal pain. *Archives of Internal Medicine* 151:694-698.

Beckman, H. B., and Frankel, R. M. 1984. The effect of physician behavior on the collection of data. *Annals of Internal Medicine* 101:692-696.

Bergner, M. 1990. Advances in health status measurement: The potential to improve experimental and non-experimental data collection. In: A. C. Gelijns, ed. *Medical Innovation at the Crossroads.* Vol. 1, *Modern Methods of Clinical Investigation.* Washington, D.C.: National Academy Press, pp. 23-32.

Berwick, D. M., Godfrey, A. B., and Roessner, J. 1990. *Curing Health Care.* San Francisco: Jossey-Bass Publishers.

Brody, H. 1980. *Placebos and the Philosophy of Medicine.* Chicago: University of Chicago Press.

Brody, H. 1982. The lie that heals: The ethics of giving placebos. *Annals of Internal Medicine* 97:112-118.

Bunker, J. P. 1990. The selection of endpoints in evaluative research. In: A. C. Gelijns, ed. *Medical Innovation at the Crossroads.* Vol. 1, *Modern Methods of Clinical Investigation.* Washington, D.C.: National Academy Press, pp. 16-22.

Bursztajn, H. J., Feinbloom, R. I., Hamm, R. M., and Brodsky, A. 1990. *Medical Choices, Medical Chances.* New York: Routledge.

Byar, D. P., Schoenfeld, D. A., Green, S. B., Amato, D. A., Davis, R., De Gruttola, V., et al. 1990. Design considerations for AIDS trials. *New England Journal of Medicine* 323:1343-1348.

Calkins, D. R., Rubenstein, L. V., Cleary, P. D., Davies, A. R., Jette, A. M., Fink, A., et al. 1991. Failure of physicians to recognize functional disability in ambulatory patients. *Annals of Internal Medicine* 114:451-454.

Carette, S., Marcoux, S., Truchon, R., Grondin, C., Gagnon, J., Allard, Y., et al. 1991. A controlled trial of corticosteroid injections into facet joints for chronic low back pain. *New England Journal of Medicine* 325:1000-1007.

Cleary, P. D., Edgman-Levitan, S., Roberts, M., Moloney, T. W., McMullen, W., Walker, J. D., et al. 1991. Patients report about their hospital care: A national survey. *Health Affairs* 10(4):254-267.

Cohen, V. 1991. Death rates in hospitals: What the new government figures mean. *Washington Post Health*, May 28, 1991, pp. 10-12.

Cole, H. M., and Wentz, A. C. 1991. A *Journal of the American Medical Association* theme issue on women's health: Call for papers. *Journal of the American Medical Association* 266:568.

Connelly, J. E., Philbrick, I. T., Smith, G. R., Jr., Kaiser, D. L., and Wymer, A. 1989. Health perceptions of primary care patients and their influence on health care utilization. *Medical Care* 27:S99-S109.

Deyo, R. A. 1991a. Fads in the treatment of low back pain. *New England Journal of Medicine* 325:1039-1040.

Deyo, R. A. 1991b. The quality of life, research, and care (editorial). *Annals of Internal Medicine* 114:695-697.

Eddy, D. M. 1984. Variations in physician practice: The role of uncertainty. *Health Affairs* 3(2):74-89.

Eddy, D. M. 1990. Clinical decision making: From theory to practice. I. The challenge. *Journal of the American Medical Association* 263:287-290.

Eddy, D. M., and Billings, J. 1988. The quality of medical evidence: Implications for quality of care. *Health Affairs* 7(1):19-32.

Ellwood, P. M. 1988. Outcomes management: A technology of patient experience. *New England Journal of Medicine* 318:1549-1556.

Engel, G. L. 1977. The need for a new medical model: A challenge for biomedicine. *Science* 196:129-136.

Engel, G. L. 1981. The clinical application of the bio-psychosocial model. *Journal of Medicine and Philosophy* 6:101-123.

Engel, G. L. 1988. How much longer must medicine's science be bound by a seventeenth-century world view? In: K. L. White, ed. *The Task of Medicine*. Menlo Park, Calif.: Henry J. Kaiser Family Foundation, pp. 113-136.

Everitt, D. E., Avorn, J., and Baker, M. W. 1990. Clinical decision making in the evaluation and treatment of insomnia. *American Journal of Medicine* 89:357-362.

Feinstein, A. R. 1983. An additional basic science for clinical medicine: IV. The development of clinimetrics. *Annals of Internal Medicine* 99:843-848.

Feinstein, A. R. 1987. The intellectual crisis in clinical science: Medaled models and muddled mettle. *Perspectives in Biology and Medicine* 30:215-230.

Fishman, S. 1988. *A Bomb in the Brain*. New York: Charles Scribner's Sons.

Foucault, M. 1975. *The Birth of the Clinic: An Archaeology of Medical Perception*. New York: Vintage Books.

Fowler, F. J., Jr., Wennberg, J. E., Timothy, R. P., Barry, M. J., Mulley, A. G., Jr., and Hanley, D. 1988. Symptom status and quality of life following prostatectomy. *Journal of the American Medical Association* 259:3018-3022.

Fox, P. 1989. From senility to Alzheimer's disease: The rise of the Alzheimer's disease movement. *Milbank Quarterly* 67:58-102.

Frank, A. W. 1991. *At the Will of the Body*. Boston: Houghton Mifflin.

Friedman, G. 1988. Home sweet hospital. *HealthWeek*, October 17, pp. 17-21.

Friedman, G. 1989. Outcomes study incorporates quality-of-life measures. *HealthWeek*, August 28, p. 4.

Fumento, M. 1990. *The Myth of Heterosexual AIDS*. New York: Basic Books.

Gadow, S. 1982. Body and self: A dialectic. In: V. Kestenbaum, ed. *The Humanity of the Ill*. Knoxville: University of Tennessee Press.

Gelijns, A. C. 1990. Comparing the development of drugs, devices, and clinical procedures. In: A. C. Gelijns, ed. *Medical Innovation at the Crossroads*. Vol. 1, *Modern Methods of Clinical Investigation*. Washington, D.C.: National Academy Press, pp. 147-201.

Gelijns, A. C., and Thier, S. O. 1990. Medical technology: An introduction to the innovation-evaluation nexus. In: A. C. Gelijns, ed. *Medical Innovation at the Crossroads*. Vol. 1, *Modern Methods of Clinical Investigation*. Washington, D.C.: National Academy Press, pp. 1-15.

Ginzberg, E., ed. 1991. *Health Services Research*. Cambridge, Mass.: Harvard University Press.

Ginzburg, E., and Lee, P. R. 1991. Physician payment. In: E. Ginzberg, ed. *Health Services Research*. Cambridge, Mass.: Harvard University Press.

Green, J. A. 1988. Minimizing malpractice risks by role clarification. *Annals of Internal Medicine* 109:234-241.

Greenfield, S., Kaplan, S. H., Ware, J. E., Jr., Yano, E. M., and Frank, H. J. L. 1988. Patient participation in medical care: Effects on blood sugar control and quality of life in diabetes. *Journal of General Internal Medicine* 3:448-457.

Hall, J. A., Epstein, A. M., and McNeil, B. J. 1989. Multi-dimensionality of health status in an elderly population. *Medical Care* 27:S168-S177.

Halm, E. A., and Gelijns, A. C. 1991. An introduction to the changing economics of technological innovation in medicine. In: A. C. Gelijns and E. A. Halm, eds. *Medical Innovation at the Crossroads*. Vol. 2, *The Changing Economics of Medical Technology*. Washington, D.C.: National Academy Press, pp. 1-20.

Hamburg, M. A., and Fauci, A. S. 1989. AIDS: The challenge to biomedical research. *Daedalus* 118(2):19-39.

Harris, Louis, and Associates, Inc. 1989. The Picker/Commonwealth Patient-Centered Care Survey. Study no. 884027.

Healy, B. 1991a. Women's health, public welfare (editorial). *Journal of the American Medical Association* 266:566-568.

Healy, B. 1991b. The Yentl syndrome (editorial). *New England Journal of Medicine* 325:274-276.

Heisenberg, W. 1958. *Physics and Philosophy, The Revolution in Modern Science*. New York: Harper Collins. Quoted in Engel, G. L. 1988. How much longer must medicine's science be bound by a seventeenth-century world view? In: K. L. White, ed. *The Task of Medicine*. Menlo Park, Calif.: Henry J. Kaiser Family Foundation.

Hellman, S., and Hellman, D. S. 1991. Of mice but not men: Problems of the randomized clinical trial. *New England Journal of Medicine* 324:1585-1589.

James, T. M. 1988. Cascades, collusions, and conflicts in cardiology (editorial). *Journal of the American Medical Association* 259:2454-2455.

Kaplan, S. H., Greenfield, S., and Ware, J. E., Jr. 1989. Assessing the effects of physician-patient interactions on the outcomes of chronic disease. *Medical Care* 27:S110-S127.

Katz, J. 1984. *The Silent World of Doctor and Patient*. New York: Free Press.

Kessler, D. A. 1989. The regulation of investigational drugs. *New England Journal of Medicine* 320:281-288.

Knox, R. A. 1991. Critiquing hospital care. *Boston Globe: The Good Health Magazine*. October 16.

Lasagna, L. 1989. Congress, the FDA, and new drug development: Before and after 1962. *Perspectives in Biology and Medicine* 32:322-343.

Lewin, T. 1987. Hospitals pitch harder for patients. *New York Times*, May 10.

Lohr, K. N., ed. 1992. Fostering the Application of Health Status Measures in Clinical Settings: Proceedings of a Conference. *Medical Care Supplement* 30: MS1-MS294.

Mairs, N. 1990. *Carnal Acts*. New York: Harper Collins Publishers.

McWhinney, I. R. 1988. Through clinical method to a more humanistic medicine. In: K. L. White, ed. *The Task of Medicine*. Menlo Park, Calif.: Henry J. Kaiser Family Foundation.

Merck Manual of Diagnosis and Therapy. 15th ed. 1987. Rahway, N.J.: Merck Sharp & Dohme Research Laboratories.

Merigan, T. C. 1990. You can teach an old dog new tricks: How AIDS trials are pioneering new strategies. *New England Journal of Medicine* 323:1341-1343.

Mold, J. M., and Stein, H. F. 1986. The cascade effect in the clinical care of patients. *New England Journal of Medicine* 314:512-514.

Moloney, T. W., and Paul, B. 1991a. The consumer movement takes hold in medical care. *Health Affairs* 10(4):268-279.

Moloney, T. W., and Paul, B. 1991b. Do Patients' Perceptions Really Matter? Report to the Board of Directors of The Commonwealth Fund. July 9.

Mulley, A. G., Jr. 1990. Medical decision making and practice variation. In: T. F. Anderson and G. M. Mooney, eds. *The Challenges of Medical Practice Variation.* London: Macmillan, pp. 59-75.

Murphy, E. *The Logic of Medicine.* Baltimore, Md.: Johns Hopkins University Press.

Murphy, R. F. 1987. *The Body Silent.* New York: Henry Holt and Company.

Nelson, E. C. 1991. Quarterly letter to HCA hospitals using HQT. Hospital Corporation of America, Nashville, Tenn. May 3.

Nelson, E. C., Hays, R. D., Larson, C., and Batalden, P. B. 1989. The patient judgment system: Reliability and validity. *Journal of Quality Assurance/Quarterly Review Bulletin* 15:185-191.

Nelson, E. C., Larson, C., and Batalden, P. B. 1990. *Voice of the Customer: Report No. 2.* Nashville, Tenn.: Hospital Corporation of America.

New York Times. 1986. Hospitals, competing for scarce patients, turn to advertising. April 20.

Nightingale, S. L. 1987. From the Food and Drug Administration: Treatment use and sale of investigational drugs. *Journal of the American Medical Association* 257:1858.

Oates, J. A., and Wood, A. J. J. 1989. Editorial: The regulation of discovery and drug development (editorial). *New England Journal of Medicine* 320:311-312.

O'Connor, F. 1956. Quoted in: Stone, J. *In the Country of Hearts.* 1990. New York: Delacorte Press.

Odegaard, C. E. 1986. *Dear Doctor.* Menlo Park, Calif.: Henry J. Kaiser Family Foundation.

Peabody, F. W. 1927. The care of the patient. *Journal of the American Medical Association* 88:877-882.

Physician Payment Review Commission. 1990. *Annual Report to Congress, 1990.* Washington, D.C.: The Commission.

Physician Payment Review Commission. 1991. *Annual Report to Congress, 1991.* Washington, D.C.: The Commission.

President's Commission for the Study of Ethical Problems in Medicine and Biomedical Research. 1982. *Making Health Care Decisions: The Ethical and Legal Implications of Informed Consent in the Patient-Practitioner Relationship.* Washington, D.C.: U.S. Government Printing Office.

Preston, T. A. 1986. *The Clay Pedestal.* New York: Charles Scribner's Sons.

Reiser, S. J. 1987. *Medicine and the Reign of Technology.* New York: Cambridge University Press.

Robinson, J. C., and H. S. Luft. 1987. Competition and the cost of hospital care, 1972 to 1982. *Journal of the American Medical Association* 257:3241-3245.

Rosenbaum, E. E. 1988. *A Taste of My Own Medicine.* New York: Random House.

Rothman, D. J., and Edgar, H. 1990. Drug approval and AIDS: Benefits for the elderly. *Health Affairs* 9(3):123-130.

Sacks, O. 1973. Preface to the original edition. In: *Awakenings.* 1987. New York: Summit Books, pp. ix-xi.

Sacks, O. 1984. *A Leg To Stand On.* New York: Summit Books.

Seldin, D. W. 1981. Presidential address: The boundaries of medicine. *Transactions of the Association of American Physicians* 94:lxxv-lxxxvi.

Smith, T. 1983. Questions on clinical trials (editorial). *British Medical Journal* 287:569. Quoted in Deyo, R. A. 1991. The quality of life, research, and care (editorial). *Annals of Internal Medicine* 114:695-697.

Southern Surgeons Club. 1991. A prospective analysis of 1,518 laparoscopic cholecystectomies. *New England Journal of Medicine* 324:1073-1078.

Spiro, H. M. 1986. *Doctors, Patients, and Placebos.* New Haven, Conn.: Yale University Press.

Starr, P. 1982. *The Social Transformation of American Medicine*. New York: Basic Books.

Stewart, A. L., Greenfield, S., Hays, R. D., Wells, K., Rogers, W. H., Berry, S. D., et al. 1989. Functional status and well-being of patients with chronic conditions. *Journal of the American Medical Association* 262:907-913.

Stewart, A. L., and Ware, J. E., Jr., eds. 1992 forthcoming. *Measuring Behavioral Function and Well-Being: The Medical Outcomes Study Approach*. Durham, N.C.: Duke University Press.

Stipp, D. 1991. Harvard HMO's Thomas Pyle resigns in row with doctors over management. *Wall Street Journal*, November 22.

Thompson, L. 1990. New ways to get medicine into the body. *Washington Post: Health*, October 2.

Toombs, S. K. 1987. The meaning of illness: A phenomenological approach to the patient-physician relationship. *Journal of Medicine and Philosophy* 12:219-240.

Toombs, S. K. 1988. Illness and the paradigm of lived body. *Theoretical Medicine* 9:202-226.

Toombs, S. K. 1989. Review of J. H. Buchanan's *Patient Encounters: The Experience of Disease*. *New Physician*, October.

Toombs, S. K. 1990. The temporality of illness: Four levels of experience. *Theoretical Medicine* 11:227-241.

Toombs, S. K. 1991. The body in multiple sclerosis: A patient's perspective. In: D. Leder, ed. *The Body in Medical Thought and Practice*. Norwell, Mass.: Kluwer Academic Publishers.

Toombs, S. K. 1992. *The Meaning of Illness: A Phenomenological Approach to the Patient-Physician Relationship* (see especially Chapter 3). Norwell, Mass.: Kluwer Academic Publishers.

U.S. plans a vast study on women's health. 1991. *New York Times*, April 20.

Ware, J. E., Jr. Quoted in Friedman, G. 1989. Outcomes study incorporates quality-of-life measures. *HealthWeek*, August 28, p. 4.

Ware, J. E., Jr. 1989. Comments on the conference on health status assessment. *Medical Care* 27:S286-S290.

Ware, J. E., Jr. 1990. Measuring patient function and well-being: Some lessons from the Medical Outcomes Study. In: K. A. Heithoff, and K. N. Lohr, eds. *Effectiveness and Outcomes in Health Care*. Washington, D.C.: National Academy Press, pp. 107-119.

Wells, K. B., Hays, R. D., Burnam, A., Rogers, W., Greenfield, S., and Ware, J. E., Jr. 1989a. Detection of depressive disorder for patients receiving prepaid or fee-for-service care. *Journal of the American Medical Association* 262:3298-3302.

Wells, K. B., Stewart, A., Hays, R. D., Burnam, A., Rogers, W., Daniels, M., et al. 1989b. The functioning and well-being of depressed patients. *Journal of the American Medical Association* 262:914-919.

Wolfe, B. M., Gardiner, B., and Frey, C. F. 1991. Laparoscopic cholecystectomy: A remarkable development. *Journal of the American Medical Association* 265:1573-1574.

Young, F. E., Norris, J. A., Levitt, J. A., and Nightingale, S. L. 1988. The FDA's new procedures for the use of investigational drugs in treatment. *Journal of the American Medical Association* 259:2267-2270.

Zucker, A. 1981. Holism and reductionism: A view from genetics. *Journal of Medicine and Philosophy* 6(2):149-150. Quoted in L. Foss and K. Rothenberg. 1987. *The Second Medical Revolution*. Boston: New Science Library/Shambala.

Part VI
Implications for Innovators

12

Managed Care and
Pharmaceutical Innovation

Frederick W. Telling

The many strong managed health care systems that emerged in the United States during the 1980s, along with federal policy changes that affect the economics of the pharmaceutical industry, are having a significant impact on industry strategies for innovation. This paper describes typical new practices and three important effects of those practices on industry operations: (1) current gatekeeping methods have altered pharmaceutical use by health care providers; (2) such controls diminish a research-based company's potential sales revenue to support innovation; and (3) the changing health care environment is altering pharmaceutical research strategies and will affect the spectrum and characteristics of drugs available in the future. These practices also lead to new policy issues relating to the growing emphasis on outcomes research and to the increasing restrictions on the dissemination of information about drugs—issues that the United States must address if its pharmaceutical industry is to remain competitive.

Three recurrent themes are central to these matters.

1. *Medical innovation is expensive.* Pharmaceutical innovation appears to be the most costly and uncertain of all efforts to develop new medical technologies. Recent studies based on a cohort of products that were first tested in humans between 1970 and 1982 have shown that research and development (R&D) for each innovative new drug (new chemical entity)

brought to the U.S. market takes 12 years and costs, on average, $231 million (in 1987 dollars; DiMasi et al., 1991). Evidence indicates that the costs associated with more recent R&D are substantially higher. The economic burden of paying for this innovation, along with the benefits of the technology, now rests squarely on countries whose health care systems are receptive to technology.

2. *Third parties are intervening in health care decisions.* Third-party payers in both the public and private sectors of the United States are moving toward the interventionist policies of health care regulators in Europe (Burstall, 1991). In the case of pharmaceuticals, the controls imposed by payers produce both economic and bureaucratic disincentives to innovation. Such controls are mediated through a diverse variety of mechanisms, which are described more fully below. Unlike Europe, however, where government is the payer of care and the promoter of industrial strength, most payers in the United States have no direct responsibility for the success of the industries that produce these products.

3. *Cost is becoming a dominant factor in the decisions of third-party payers and appears to be replacing patient benefit as the principal factor for determining whether an innovative technology is adopted and used.* Although third-party payers rightly emphasize the importance of data on both health and economic outcomes to justify the acceptance of a technology, generally, they have not shared the responsibility for evaluative research to generate such data.

MANAGED CARE PRACTICES, GATEKEEPING, AND HEALTH CARE DELIVERY

Earlier chapters in this volume describe the evolution of U.S. health care policy and its economic consequences. Projections of 1992 health care expenditures in this country, well fueled on both the demand and supply sides, are $817 billion, or 14 percent of the gross national product (GNP; U.S. Department of Commerce, 1992). Most of this expense is paid by government and by private employer-funded benefit plans. However, coverage and reimbursement across the spectrum of health services vary widely. In 1990, patients paid about 5 percent of hospital care directly out of their own pockets; they paid about 19 percent of physician costs and 74 percent of prescription drug expenses (NCPA/Fiscal Associates, 1990). Despite the relatively small portion—5 percent—of total U.S. health care costs represented by pharmaceuticals (HCFA, Office of the Actuary, 1992) and the limited reimbursement of pharmaceutical charges by institutional payers, the pervasive concerns of such payers about health care costs have nonetheless affected pharmaceutical usage (Grabowski, 1991).

Widening Constraints on Health Care Services

Earlier in this volume, Soper and Ferriss, Wagner, and Welch and Fisher describe the evolution of public and private benefit plans from essentially passive payers to active purchasers of health care. In this new role, payers explicitly seek to constrain both the price and the intensity (volume) of health care services. Health maintenance organizations (HMOs), which integrate the delivery and financing of comprehensive health services, have been the main innovators in devising the cost-control methodologies that have come to be called managed care. The diffusion of the concepts of managed care from HMOs, which cover about 15 percent of the population, to traditional indemnity plans has occurred rapidly and without major fanfare or debate. These techniques now promise to pervade all U.S. health benefit plans within this decade.

The objective of managed care is to discourage unnecessary and inappropriate medical services without jeopardizing necessary, high-quality care. In a broad sense, managed care employs various techniques and degrees of third-party influence to affect the patient's choice of health care provider and the pricing, type, and volume of the provider's goods and services. As a result, it has acquired the label of *gatekeeper*. Managed care represents a fundamental structural shift to a health care delivery system in which the judgments of third-party payers are interposed in traditional physician-patient decision making.

Pressures on Drug Costs

The cost-containment tools of managed care generally comprise coverage design and administration, payment limits, and selective contracting with providers of health care services and goods. To evaluate the potential applicability of such techniques to pharmaceutical selection and usage, it is important to understand the economic structure of the U.S. pharmaceutical market and the American approach to pharmaceutical cost containment as lucidly described by Grabowski (1991). Enactment of the Drug Price Competition and Patent Term Restoration Act in 1984 facilitated the transfer of inventors' intellectual property by establishing a regulatory framework to expedite the marketing of generic copies of a drug. Frequently, generic copies are ready for marketing on the expiration date of the innovator's patent (plus the time extension, if any, provided by the terms of the act). The principal economic consequence of this policy is to oblige the innovator to attempt to recoup all of the costs of research, development, and market diffusion of the new product during the considerably shortened period of patent exclusivity; this period must be used as well to provide adequate returns to shareholders and to invest in future products. Wholesale prices of generic copies can be much lower than that of the original product because generics are brought to market generally with development investments of less than $1 million (less than 0.5 percent of the innovator's cost) and few, if any, market diffusion expenses (because the innovator's knowledge contribution has already been transferred).

The price differentials between patented, single-source pharmaceuticals and their generic counterparts have created a two-tiered market for pharmaceuticals whose patents have expired. Not surprisingly, substantial market shares have shifted to generics, in both institutional settings, where the influence of third-party payers dominates, and in outpatient dispensing, where generics provide attractive profit margins to the retail pharmacy (Masson and Steiner, 1985; Bloom et al., 1986). The shift is so dramatic that sales of the innovator's product have been found to decrease by 50 percent within 2 years of the introduction of the generic competitor (Grabowski and Vernon, 1990).

The attractive price differentials provided by generics are an obvious target for managed care policies related to pharmaceutical acceptance and usage. Among the drug substitution techniques that have been adopted extensively by public and private payers are limited formularies that typically favor generics and impose barriers to the inclusion of single-source pharmaceuticals; mandatory substitution of a generic when a branded pharmaceutical is prescribed; therapeutic substitution of a different but therapeutically similar drug when a single-source pharmaceutical is prescribed; and step-care protocols that typically require the trial of one or more less expensive medications before a more expensive, single-source drug may be used. By their nature these practices favor the use of old therapies rather than new innovative drugs and may harm the quality of patient care (Oster et al., 1987).

A variety of ancillary techniques are frequently applied to reinforce these policies for pharmaceutical cost containment in managed care settings. They include minimization of the value of differential benefits in patient subgroups, exclusion of non-approved uses, incorporation of drug reimbursement in prospectively fixed payments for physician and hospital services, direct drug purchasing using competitive bidding, pharmacy capitation payments, drug utilization review, and, more recently, inhibition of physicians' access to new product information from traditional sources.

The Unknown Effects of Managed Care

Unfortunately, as yet only limited information is available about the effects of managed care gatekeeping on health outcomes, health care innovation, and health care costs. Where the focus of managed care is solely on the short-term control of drug costs and subsequent benefit payments, the result may be diminished quality of care, increases in the total cost of care (e.g., because of the use of less effective medications or procedures), or both. For example, Soumerai and colleagues (1991) recently reported a twofold increase in nursing home admission rates in a New Hampshire Medicaid population following the imposition of a limit on outpatient dispensing of drugs. When the limit was removed, drug use and admission rates returned to their prelimit levels, but most of the patients admitted during the period of the restriction remained in nursing homes. The cost of the presumed excess institutionalization was estimated to far exceed the savings ascribed to the limit on prescribing. In another instance, Sisk and coworkers (1991) have described the detrimental effects of a restrictive Medicare policy on drug treatment of anemia in dialysis patients.

The development of sound policies for pharmaceutical use obviously demands a great deal of medical and economic information that often is not available. Managed care firms may have both the data and the incentive to help fill these information voids. An interesting example of such a study appeared early in 1990; based on 1987 data, it was designed as a comprehensive empirical comparison of prescription drug use in managed care plans and traditional benefit plans. The study found that HMO enrollees had a substantially higher rate of prescription drug use than those in traditional benefit plans. About 14 percent of the claims in the traditional plan were for generic products, whereas the average for generic claims across the HMOs was about 35 percent. Moreover, there were significant, unexplained variations in prescription drug use among the HMOs, suggesting the persistence of varying physician practice patterns under managed care (Weiner et al., 1991).

MANAGED CARE GATEKEEPING: EFFECTS ON THE PHARMACEUTICAL INDUSTRY AND PHARMACEUTICAL INNOVATION

Pressure on Resources for R&D

The changes in the U.S. pharmaceutical marketplace that are described above and by Grabowski (1991) have profound economic consequences for the research-based pharmaceutical firm. The shortened commercial life span of single-source pharmaceutical products reduces the cash flow available to the firm to fund the increasingly expensive ongoing R&D needed to replenish its constantly eroding product portfolio. And even this growing investment in R&D is not being translated into a correspondingly larger number of new drugs. Much of the added investment is directed toward meeting increased regulatory requirements that prolong the drug development cycle.

Payer strategies for containment of pharmaceutical costs powerfully amplify these economic effects and make it even more difficult for a firm to achieve a satisfactory return on its investment. For older, branded drugs, the strategies accelerate the decline in their market share; for new, innovative drugs, they both diminish pricing flexibility and impede the diffusion and use of new products. For example, a study of Medicaid formulary practice has revealed delays of as long as 4 years in the acceptance of new products for reimbursement; such delays further shorten the commercial life of the product. Therapeutic substitution and step-care protocols present additional barriers to the diffusion of new pharmaceuticals and reduce the economic return to the innovator.

Pressure for Products with Well-Defined Costs and Benefits

New practices of third-party payers have contributed to the development of a broader conceptualization of outcomes research—that is, health *and* economic outcomes research that systematically assesses the impact of an intervention on such measures as cost, quality of life, functional status, and patient satisfaction. Although the measurement of health outcomes has been carried out in the past, combining it with economic outcomes, in which the consequences of health care interventions are compared with their costs, is a more recent practice. Such research can be expected to increase our understanding of the effectiveness of alternative interventions, bring about better decision making by physicians and patients, and, more controversially, lead to the development of practice standards to guide physicians and aid payers in optimizing the use of resources. The growing importance of economic analysis of pharmaceuticals is reflected by the more than 680 articles published on the subject in 1990, a 25-fold increase since 1966, and a new journal, *PharmacoEconomics*, beginning publication in 1992 (Eisenberg, 1992).

For pharmaceutical companies, the implications of the new focus on outcomes research are quite clear. More elaborate and costly clinical studies must be carried out to provide the persuasive case needed for the new drug to be accepted by gatekeepers who at the same time will be putting pressure on the prices of innovative drugs. Such studies typically require a minimum of many years, thousands of patients, and tens of millions of dollars. Those innovators who can introduce valuable new modalities that are also cost saving will have significant potential for success. However, firms offering products that increase costs will need to demonstrate a more favorable health outcome before the product is considered for use and reimbursement.

In addition, pharmaceutical cost-containment strategies have important second-order economic effects that influence the R&D strategies of the innovator. As discussed later, these barriers to the entry and use of a new drug in the marketplace drive the innovator toward more exploratory, and therefore higher risk, research projects in the quest for breakthrough innovations.

Pressure to Limit the Transfer of Information on Drugs

Once an innovative new product reaches the market, increasing pressures restrict the diffusion of information about its benefits. The Food and Drug Administration's (FDA) recent restrictions on industry's support of scientific symposia and physicians' involvement in disseminating new knowledge are a case in point. Some managed care systems that do not permit the dissemination of industry-sponsored information are troubling not only because of the adversarial relationship of innovators and users that such measures suggest but also because of their potentially negative impact on patient care.

The practices of Kaiser Permanente, the nation's largest HMO system with more than 6 million enrolled members, illustrate how the diffusion and use of new drugs can be limited. In addition to implementing therapeutic substitution and step-care protocols common to many managed care systems, Kaiser management recently began to severely limit contact of the HMO's physicians with pharmaceutical sales representatives. Practices that restrict the type of product information that can be communicated, that limit the access of sales representatives to facilities, that counter the scientific information provided by companies and prohibit the communication of scientific information about nonformulary products, and that do not allow physicians to attend industry symposia present additional barriers to the diffusion of new pharmaceuticals into the market. In no instance has there been an assessment of the effects of such practices; nevertheless, other managed care systems are adopting similar restrictive policies.

Increased Economic Risk for Pharmaceutical Innovation

A substantial body of empirical evidence from economic studies of the pharmaceutical industry is entirely consistent with the expected effects of the market forces just described. Particularly striking is Grabowski and Vernon's (1990) finding that fewer than one-third of the innovative new pharmaceuticals (new chemical entities) introduced into the U.S. market in the 1970s had a positive return on the average R&D investment (including the cost of capital). Furthermore, during the 1980s, as more foreign-based pharmaceutical companies have produced world-class products, U.S.-based companies have experienced declines in their U.S. market share for the economically most important innovative new drugs, compared with the shares they maintained for such drugs in the 1970s (Althuis, 1992). Global economic pressure on the industry is also fostering closer relationships based on the scientific and competitive expertise of individual firms. U.S. firms supported the costs of licensing many of the top innovative new drugs in the 1980s and executed the clinical studies required to bring them to the U.S. market. Also tightening the squeeze on economic return is the dramatic increase in the industry's R&D expenditures from $2 billion in 1980 to $9.2 billion in 1991 (PMA, 1991), in the face of a more competitive environment and obvious financial distress in the case of some firms. Notable also is the rapidly increasing share earmarked for clinical R&D (phases 1, 2, and 3): 17 percent of R&D expenditures in 1979 but 27 percent in 1989 (PMA, 1991). Partly in response to these trends, an increasing amount of clinical research by U.S. companies is moving overseas where large multicenter trials are often easier and less costly to conduct (Gelijns, 1990).

The economics of pharmaceutical innovation are likely to become increasingly strained as the techniques of managed care become more stringent and are applied more broadly. The implications of this trend for the future of the industry may well be prefigured by the consolidation that has already occurred both explicitly, in the form of the mergers of world-class firms, which have been seen at unparalleled levels over the past 5 years, and implicitly, through the now widespread practice of two or more firms "co-marketing" newly approved pharmaceutical products. Other aspects of industry's response to the changing economic environment are becoming apparent as well. First, as discussed in the next section, research-based firms are taking a number of steps to adapt their R&D programs to the realities of the new pharmaceutical marketplace. Second, the industry is facing new policy issues that must be addressed soon if the United States is to remain the world leader in pharmaceutical innovation. These issues are discussed later in this paper.

PHARMACEUTICAL RESEARCH STRATEGIES FOR A CHANGING HEALTH CARE ENVIRONMENT

The Promising Technology Base

Before turning to the research strategies that appear to be industry's responses to the new market factors, it is important to recognize that contemporary pharmaceutical R&D is being influenced by profound developments in science and technology. Advances in the understanding of biology at the molecular level and in the power of scientific instrumentation, coupled with enhanced computer capabilities, have empowered researchers in their search for new drugs. The most important consequence of this empowerment has been the research scientist's growing ability to understand physiological and pathological processes in molecular terms and to synthe-size receptors and create biological models of disease phenomena.   An additional bonus for researchers is the assistance of computers in thinking through sophisticated concepts by employing complex theoretical analyses that were simply impossible to carry out even a decade ago.

As a result, the empirical approaches of past decades have been largely displaced by more rational approaches to drug design. Contemporary drug research focuses on understanding the biology of disease and intervening in the sequence of specific biological events that characterize a disease in order to treat it. Experimental drugs are now designed, or efficiently screened (tested in large numbers), or both, to capitalize on their ability to interact with bioreceptors that have high probabilities of being therapeutically relevant.

This change in research focus is well illustrated by the explicit mecha-nistic characterization of the new drugs that started to emerge in sizable numbers in the 1980s: for example, angiotensin-converting enzyme (ACE) inhibitors, calcium-channel blockers, histamine H-2 receptor antagonists, and so forth. Scientists' improved understanding of disease mechanisms and processes is opening up new drug discovery approaches to attack dis-eases and conditions—such as osteoporosis, Alzheimer's disease, memory loss, migraine, and depression—that in earlier decades could not be system-atically addressed through pharmaceutical research.

The 1990s are likely to see a blossoming of three major trends in phar-maceutical innovation, the products of which began to emerge in sizable numbers in the 1980s. First, one can expect an even more diverse set of new small-molecule drugs that modulate disease by an understood mecha-nism—for example, serotonin re-uptake blockers, aldose reductase inhibi-tors, and immune stimulators. Second, the new biotechnology, which makes possible the synthesis of complex proteins, will offer a broader array of such complex large-molecule drugs. Both of these approaches will be used to produce an increasing proportion of drugs to treat chronic or metabolic diseases, to develop treatments for long-term complications of disease, and to offer significant steps toward medications for the prevention of disease. Third, the utility of both large- and small-molecule drugs will be amplified by promising improvements in drug delivery technology for the sustained release of drugs, for the absorption of protein drugs, and for drugs attached to lyposomes, which are designed to deliver the drug to a specific site and thereby reduce side effects.

In sum, the research-based pharmaceutical industry now has in place the technical capability with which to tackle the more intractable diseases and therapeutic needs that up to now have not been amenable to drug inter-vention. If this proves to be the case, it is a timely development indeed, since the new market of the 1990s and beyond may only be accessible to new pharmaceuticals that serve unmet needs. Additionally, such innovation offers the potential to directly address the current growth in health care costs by eliminating the necessity for whole areas of care (Brown and Luce, 1990; Brown et al., 1991).

Enhanced Focus on Innovation

The development of a modern drug is one of the most complex processes undertaken by any industry. Drug discovery projects that are initiated today must produce a product to meet the standards, conditions, and needs of the year 2000 and beyond. The great financial investment that is now needed for successful pharmaceutical R&D (possibly in excess of $400 million for each new chemical entity), the dramatically intensified competition at home and abroad, and the significantly increased U.S. preoccupation with health care cost containment are placing significant pressure on drug industry managers who are responsible for product innovation. By the year 2000, the technology gatekeepers will be less tolerant of imitative drugs that fail to offer added value. If an innovative firm is to compete, it must succeed in discovering new drugs whose value and effectiveness are demonstrably greater than those offered by other therapies. The degree to which a firm can convince gatekeepers that it has achieved these ends will be an important determinant of how quickly and easily the new product can enter the market.

The market environment, which is increasingly influenced by managed care gatekeepers, is already forcing pharmaceutical research managers to evaluate alternative discovery risk options carefully and, in some cases, to shift significantly the balance of their research portfolios in terms of the types of drugs and diseases toward which R&D resources will be directed. Some key considerations in today's discovery research strategies include the following:

• *New disease targets.* It is reasonable to anticipate a relative deemphasis of research in therapeutic categories that will be well served by generic drugs; the generic armamentarium for such conditions as gastric and duodenal ulcer and essential hypertension will be greatly expanded as a result of patent expirations in the mid- to late 1990s. On the basis of known patent expiration dates, it is easy to project the timing of generic entry as much as a decade in advance. When such an entry occurs, the gatekeepers' criteria for successful entry of new, costly, single-source medications in that category will be formidable indeed.

The new knowledge of molecular biology, coupled with commodity-like competition in old therapeutic areas, makes it reasonable to anticipate research emphasis on new drugs that provide added value, that is, drugs for therapeutic targets that are not currently amenable to treatment and for disease targets that have only limited existing therapy in terms of effectiveness, tolerance, toxicity, convenience, or cost. Consistent with the new emphasis on systemwide optimization, drug research has been actively seeking pharmaceutical alternatives to high-cost surgical procedures (e.g., benign prostatic hypertrophy, angioplasty) and costly chronic care (e.g., osteoporosis, Alzheimer's disease).

• *Well-differentiated, value-added drugs.* This phrase characterizes the major strategy of most firms, which seeks to create highly innovative, well-differentiated new drugs with added therapeutic value that will have the least risk of incurring regulatory delay and the best chance of achieving market acceptance. A key aspect of this approach is to seek a meaningful differentiation of a potential new drug candidate early in the research process—and to drop it early in the process if such differentiation is not clear. Discovering and developing a drug of this type, however, requires expensive, highly innovative discovery research that carries the greatest chance of technology failure.

When a body of scientific knowledge crystallizes in the scientific community, a number of research groups may independently and simultaneously carry out value-added drug discovery research working from the same base of knowledge, from similar perceptions of medical need, and from a recognition of commercial opportunity. In such cases, several new but somewhat different drugs with the same therapeutic mechanism may emerge in a narrow time frame. The question is, how will the gatekeeper view them? Will all but the first be a sizable risk in terms of market acceptability?

• *"Fast-follower" drugs.* This research strategy recognizes that the first drug in a new therapeutic class is not likely to be the optimum version. Firms with the capability to quickly discover a second or third drug with a more favorable safety and efficacy profile or a more convenient route of administration may also receive a reasonable return on their R&D investment. A fast-follower has less chance of technology failure but is likely to encounter more difficulty than the initial value-added product in passing the many hurdles of regulatory and market acceptability. The "window of opportunity" for exploiting a new class of drugs in this manner is likely to narrow considerably through the 1990s. This is an unfortunate circumstance for medicine and for the patient. It will discourage the kind of incremental advances that in past decades have provided important building blocks of medical knowledge, and it will narrow the field of choice from which physicians can seek the optimum drug in a therapeutic class for a given patient.

• *Imitative drugs.* During the 1980s, the rapidly escalating costs of R&D, coupled with regulatory delays and decreasing opportunities to capture a share of the market, have significantly decreased industry research on new imitative drugs. In contemporary terminology, imitative drugs are "late followers" that chemically are closely related to their predecessors and act by the same mechanism as the original new drug, but offer no demonstrable advantages. The pressures being exerted by gatekeepers are likely to reduce the use of this approach even further, if not curtail it altogether, in the 1990s.

• *Enhanced delivery systems.* Another widely embraced R&D strategy calls for more emphasis on the development of superior delivery systems to improve the therapeutic profile of existing medicines. Such reformulated products typically meet important patient needs and enjoy a modest period of market exclusivity, based on patent or regulatory policy, thereby providing an incremental economic return to the innovator. It is reasonable to expect that most chronic-use oral drugs ultimately will be made available in a once-a-day, long-acting dosage and that a number of parenteral or injectable drugs—even proteins—eventually will be provided in practical oral forms.

Complex Development Strategies to Demonstrate Added Value

The design and execution of clinical development programs for new pharmaceuticals will become even more critical in the 1990s than they were in the past decade. Of even greater importance will be the pursuit of improved process efficiency (e.g., mega-clinical trials, computerized new drug applications) begun in the 1980s. In addition, new industry-wide clinical development strategies are emerging to deal with the more complex clinical studies needed to demonstrate outcomes.

• *Outcomes research.* Larger, more sophisticated, and more expensive clinical outcomes studies are being planned to demonstrate that, in addition to meeting regulatory requirements for safety and efficacy, a new drug has added value compared with alternative treatments. Such studies are seeking to identify those therapeutic characteristics that usefully differentiate the new drug from existing modalities and to demonstrate those differences with sufficient data to convince gatekeepers. In fact, a few recently introduced drugs seem to have been developed or marketed (or both) with considerable attention to the likely interests, and purchasing guidelines, of managed care gatekeepers.

In addition to seeking more information about the health and economic outcomes of alternative courses of care, companies are gearing up to engage in new kinds of research, including studies on patient preferences and compliance. The need to expand clinical research programs to include comparative endpoints of interest to gatekeepers will require more expensive research undertaken earlier in the R&D process than has been typical in the 1980s. The perceived potential for demonstrable benefits that will exceed costs may ultimately become a key criterion for the selection of research projects capable of producing candidates for full-scale development.

• *Collaborative studies of outcomes.* The best way to demonstrate the value of pharmaceutical innovations to prospective purchasers is through clinical trials that prove the effectiveness (utility under average conditions of use) of the innovation in the hands of typical health care providers. The new emphasis on such evidence may lead to cooperative studies with the gatekeepers themselves. One example worth watching is the 2-year-old technology assessment program of the Voluntary Hospitals of America (VHA). VHA is planning collaborative studies (e.g., to evaluate competing thrombolytic agents) to improve its recommendations on technologies and the buying decisions of its 850 member hospitals.

Research-based companies are also seeking to include their products in national outcomes studies, for example, those undertaken by the Patient Outcome Research Teams (PORTs), sponsored by the new Agency for Health Care Policy and Research. Such federal studies, however, represent only a fraction of the evaluative clinical research that is needed and that is being undertaken—which suggests the need for an effective partnership. In single-company and industry-wide or industry-buyer studies, it is reasonable to expect that research on outcomes, such as patient quality of life, will become more common and more important.

NEW POLICY ISSUES CRITICAL
TO U.S. COMPETITIVENESS IN PHARMACEUTICALS

As recently as a decade ago, American physicians were the primary arbiters of appropriate care for patients, and payers paid the claims for such care largely without questioning those decisions. However, as increasing subsidization of health care led to spiraling costs, payer-based gatekeeping arose (NCPA/Fiscal Associates, 1990). To date, the gatekeepers targeted for control those new technologies that cannot demonstrate, early on, that they are cost-effective and provide important patient benefits.

Clearly, some of the effects of the new managed care policies in regard to pharmaceutical R&D are benefits to society. They include demonstrations of cost-effectiveness and improved quality of life, and other outcomes research measures. But what about the research-based pharmaceutical industry? Is the current preoccupation with cost containment (or cost rationalization) detrimental to the strength of pharmaceutical firms? Not necessarily; an "adapt or vanish" environment (Burstall, 1991) provides powerful incentives for management to be more creative and more efficient, and industry is clearly responding. Managed care gatekeeping policies have, however, brought two new problems that must be addressed quite soon if the nation's investment in pharmaceutical innovation is to be maintained.

1. *Policies to promote collaborative outcomes research are needed.* Policies that support a collaborative, comprehensive approach to and re-

sponsibility for both evaluative research and patient care must be adopted. Such policies should promote cooperative funding of and participation and collaboration in the execution of outcomes work. To adapt Peter Hutt's earlier remarks regarding FDA (1991), managed care gatekeepers must move to a regulatory process driven by policies rather than people and must employ more "consistency, predictability [and] fairness among payers" in coverage and payment policies (Hutt, 1991, p. 175).

Today, many people and groups are interested in outcomes research, and the general expectation is that the pharmaceutical industry will unconditionally underwrite these new, sophisticated, and costly studies that payers increasingly demand as a precondition for a pharmaceutical's general use. Such an expectation is unreasonable if for no other reason than that it fails to recognize that evaluation of any medical technology takes time: adequate time is necessary to assess a technology in practical use (to gauge its effectiveness) and to determine the value of therapies that prevent or delay the onset of disease. If the time needed to complete such studies is so long that an insufficient period of market exclusivity remains after completion of the study, there is no economic incentive for the innovator to undertake the research.

We must recognize that it is not scientifically or economically possible to know everything about a new drug before it has been in wide use. Even more time is required to determine the value of therapies that seek to prevent or delay the onset of disease. Outcomes research needs to compare a spectrum of therapies—drug and non-drug, new and old. Whereas the pharmaceutical firm can and should carry out the early outcomes research on the merits of its new treatment, it is less reasonable to expect a firm to carry out lengthy studies comparing its product with a variety of alternative therapies in diverse settings—particularly if those studies cannot provide results well within the effective market life of the product.

Government agencies, on the other hand, may have a valuable role to play in data collection from both retrospective and possibly prospective clinical assessments in instances in which the number of alternatives to be studied is large and the time required for the study is long. Indeed, the National Institutes of Health (NIH) has assumed this kind of role in sponsoring or fostering collaborative studies for the general benefit of medical practice when the study design for comparing alternative therapies and therapies with novel modes of action was truly beyond the resources and interests of a single sponsor. For example, NIH has initiated the Treatment of Mild Hypertension Study (TOMHS), which compares the effects of five new and old antihypertensive agents, as well as diet, lifestyle, and placebo, in lowering blood pressure. NIH also undertook the Sorbinil Retinopathy Trial (SRT), which examined the usefulness of a new class of drug—an aldose reductase inhibitor—to prevent early-stage retinopathy, a major risk factor for blindness in diabetics. Everyone expects to benefit from this sort of outcomes research, and all should be willing to share the burden of executing the work. Any other policy can only be viewed as the establishment of barriers to technology development and innovation.

2. *The results of outcomes research should be freely communicated.* The second new problem facing the pharmaceutical industry relates to the collection and dissemination of innovation-specific information on medical therapies. Favorable findings from outcomes studies pose some as yet unresolved questions about how to disseminate scientific information to both practitioners and patients. One of the positive aspects of the health care system's current fascination with outcomes studies is that it explicitly encompasses patient-centered models of care. It then follows that product regulators (the FDA, the Health Care Financing Administration, and the Blue Cross/Blue Shield Association or Health Insurance Association of America), and especially managed care gatekeepers, should actively seek patient or care-giver input regarding newly available information to help sort out clinical alternatives and preferences. Although such a trend is being seen in some areas, the opposite is also occurring, as was discussed earlier in this paper.

Why should the patient's interest be neglected on this issue? In a time of transition from affluence to constraints and from doctor-centered decision making to payer-centered decision making—essentially, from old rules to new—is it possible to provide consumers with too much information about what is known or not known about their health care services? Yet patients are being left out of the decision-making process. Managed care is operating to make choices for them while they have little information on which to base an opinion regarding their therapeutic options. This shift is happening despite the fact that recent polls (Gallup Organization, Inc., personal communication, 1990) show a willingness on the part of patients to pay out of pocket to avoid some managed care restrictions.

SUMMARY

If the research-based pharmaceutical enterprise is to survive the transition now being seen in the U.S. health care system, society must recognize and address two pivotal issues:

1. *Innovation is expensive.* The industry probably cannot hope to spend less, but it can expect to spend better. **Interested parties—here and abroad—should be willing to seek ways in which to cooperate and share in the work and costs of broader evaluative research and innovative patient care.**

2. *Information transfer must not be impeded.* If cost (or payment level) is replacing patient benefit as the threshold criterion for the adoption

and use of innovative technologies, physicians and patients must be informed about the alternatives to these technologies and the consequences of their use. Even if a patient-centered model of care is adopted by managed care systems in the 1990s, increasingly educated and affluent consumers of services and products will expect more information about their clinical options. **National and organizational policies must promote, not retard, information sharing about technology.**

Favorable overall economic policies toward medical innovation and the implementation of managed health care across our country are critical to the future of the U.S. pharmaceutical industry. Either we as a nation make systemwide changes to better balance investment in innovation and cost constraints, or our innovative edge may be dulled by the advances of foreign competitors. Should this trend continue, we will eventually lose know-how, jobs, and profits to others, and probably end up wondering how we let these things happen. The U.S. pharmaceutical and biotechnology industry is currently strong and able to meet the challenges of improving America's health if the nation's policies provide a favorable environment in which it can succeed.

REFERENCES

Althuis, T. H. 1992. A therapeutic and economic comparison of the top innovative new drugs of the 1970s and 1980s. *Drug Information Journal* 26:279-287.

Bloom, B. S., Wierz, M. A., and Pauly, M. V. 1986. Cost and price of comparable branded and generic pharmaceuticals. *Journal of the American Medical Association* 256:2523-2530.

Brown, R. E., and Luce, B. R. 1990. *The Value of Pharmaceuticals: A Study of Selected Conditions to Measure the Contribution of Pharmaceuticals to Health Status.* Washington, D.C.: Battelle Human Affairs Research Centers. March.

Brown, R. E., Elixhauser, A., Sheingold, S., and Luce, B. R. 1991. *The Value of Pharmaceuticals: An Assessment of Future Costs for Selected Conditions.* Washington, D.C.: Battelle Human Affairs Research Centers. February.

Burstall, M. L. 1991. European policies influencing pharmaceutical innovation. In: A. C. Gelijns and E. A. Halm, eds. *Medical Innovation at the Crossroads.* Vol. 2, *The Changing Economics of Medical Technology.* Washington, D.C.: National Academy Press, pp. 123-140.

DiMasi, J. A., Hansen, R. W., Grabowski, H. G., and Lasagna, L. 1991. Cost of innovation in the pharmaceutical industry. *Journal of Health Economics* 10:107-142.

Eisenberg, J. M. 1992. Why a journal of pharmacoeconomics? *PharmacoEconomics* 1(1):2-4.

Gelijns, A. C. 1990. Appendix A: Comparing the Development of Drugs, Devices, and Clinical Procedures. In: A. C. Gelijns, ed. *Medical Innovation at the Crossroads.* Vol. 1, *Modern Methods of Clinical Investigation.* Washington, D.C.: National Academy Press, pp. 147-201.

Grabowski, H. 1991. The changing economics of pharmaceutical research and development. In: A. C. Gelijns and E. A. Halm, eds. *Medical Innovation at the Crossroads.* Vol. 2,

The Changing Economics of Medical Technology. Washington, D.C.: National Academy Press, pp. 35-52.

Grabowski, H., and Vernon, J. 1990. A new look at the returns and risks to pharmaceutical R&D. *Management Science* 36:804-821.

HCFA (Health Care Financing Administration), Office of the Actuary. 1992. Issue Brief Number 122. Cited by the Employee Benefit Research Institute. Washington, D.C. January.

Hutt, P. B. 1991. The impact of regulation and reimbursement on pharmaceutical innovation. In: A. C. Gelijns and E. A. Halm, eds. *Medical Innovation at the Crossroads.* Vol. 2, *The Changing Economics of Medical Technology.* Washington, D.C.: National Academy Press, pp. 169-180.

Masson, A., and Steiner, R. L. 1985. *Generic Substitution and Prescription Drug Prices: Economic Effects of State Drug Product Selection Laws.* Federal Trade Commission. Washington, D.C.: U.S. Government Printing Office.

NCPA (National Center for Policy Analysis)/Fiscal Associates. 1990. U.S. Medical Market Model Project. Personal communication from Gary Robbins. Dallas, Texas/Arlington, Virginia.

Oster, G., Huse, D. M., Delea, T. E., Savage, D. D., and Coldtz, G. A. 1987. Cost effectiveness of labetalol and propranolol in the treatment of hypertension among blacks. *Journal of the National Medical Association* 79:1049-1055.

PMA (Pharmaceutical Manufacturers Association). 1991. *1989-1991 Annual Survey Report.* Washington, D.C.: The Association, p. 28.

Sisk, J. E., Gianfrancesco, F. D., and Coster, J. M. 1991. Recombinant erythropoietin and Medicare payment. *Journal of the American Medical Association* 266:247-252.

Soumerai, S. B., Ross-Degnan, D., Avorn, J., McLaughlin, T. J., and Choodnovskiy, I. 1991. Effects of Medicaid drug-payment limits on admission to hospitals and nursing homes. *New England Journal of Medicine* 325:1072-1077.

U.S. Department of Commerce. 1992. Health and medical services. In: *U.S. Industrial Outlook '92: Business Forecasts for 350 Industries.* Washington, D.C.: U.S. Government Printing Office, p. 43-3.

Weiner, J. P., Lyles, A., Steinwachs, D. M., and Hall, K. C. 1991. Impact of managed care on prescription drug use. *Health Affairs* 10(1):140-154.

13

Current Strategies for the Development of Medical Devices

Ben L. Holmes

This paper discusses the impact of the payment and regulatory environment over the past quarter century on the demand for new medical devices in the United States, and the resultant changes in both the device industry and its product development strategies. It describes three distinct periods, each initiated by signal events: (1) from the start of Medicare and Medicaid in 1965 to the advent of the Device Law in 1976; (2) from 1976 to the advent of a prospective payment system (PPS) and diagnosis-related groups (DRGs) in 1983; and finally, (3) the period of payment reform, from 1983 to the present. This third period is discussed in greater detail than the others, given the changes that have been occurring in the market at this time and its increasing dynamism and complexity. The paper discusses the implications of those changes for research and development (R&D) investment over time and concludes with some observations on impediments to continued innovation.

PUBLIC POLICY AND MEDICAL DEVICES: 1965–1976

The period from 1965 to 1976 is significant in the development of the medical device industry because of the introduction of the Medicare and Medicaid programs, which stimulated an era of growth. In 1965 the medical device market was relatively small; U.S. Department of Commerce estimates put total sales at around $200 million. The health care system, which was almost entirely one of retrospective, cost-based, fee-for-service payment, directly encouraged the adoption of medical devices by providers. An enormous influx of health care dollars into the economy through Medicare and Medicaid programs provided major support to this system and further stimulated the diffusion of innovative medical devices.

In response to this growing demand and growth in the scientific and engineering knowledge base (as a result of investment in science and technology during World War II), many new devices and instruments were introduced. Classic products introduced during this period include patient monitoring systems, computerized catheterization laboratories, electrocardiogram (ECG) management systems, fetal monitors, and computed tomography (CT) scanners.

PUBLIC POLICY AND MEDICAL DEVICES: 1976–1983

The next period was one of increasing government regulation initiated by the enactment in 1976 of the Medical Device Amendments to the Food, Drug, and Cosmetic Act. The enactment of the amendments gave the government, through the Food and Drug Administration (FDA), ground-breaking authority over medical devices. They authorized the FDA to evaluate and approve new medical technologies to ensure their safety and efficacy and to assess manufacturer claims of effectiveness.

At the same time, the market was being fueled by growing national wealth, the public's belief in the products of biomedical research, and the demands of providers for new and improved devices (Shabot, 1990). This latter factor was of particular importance. Physicians, because of their training and their role as patient advocates, strive to do as much as possible for their patients. During these high-growth years, however, patients and providers alike became more insulated from the financial consequences of the physician decisions regarding appropriate health care. Payment continued to be open-ended. With few limits on the availability of funds, capital equipment purchase decisions were often based on the belief that more care was necessarily better care (Altman and Rodwin, 1988).

The period from 1976 to 1983 saw, for the first time, the appearance of several very high priced new modalities—for example, magnetic resonance imaging (MRI) systems that sold for $2 million dollars and required an additional $1 million for siting. Medical devices became increasingly sophisticated, and these kinds of major, capital-intensive health care investments were soon perceived by some to be the culprit responsible for the rising costs of health care. According to the Office of Technology Assessment, the utilization of medical technology accounted for nearly one-third of the 107 percent increase in Medicare spending per patient between 1977 and 1982 (Office of Technology Assessment, 1984).[1] With health care costs of all kinds rising, the government attempted to control this escalation by restricting the flow of capital coming into the market. States also began to look for ways to control costs, and introduced certificates of need (CON) to control the diffusion of high-tech medical equipment.

Implications for Medical Device R&D

What were the implications of these changes for the medical device industry? During this period, industrial R&D strategies remained relatively similar. In spite of government intervention, the market did not change appreciably. Government intervention in the form of FDA regulation extended the time required to bring a product to market, but not significantly. Thus, there was only modest or no decline in 1976 when the Device Amendments were implemented. In the opinion of this author, the lack of change in the market confirms that the medical device amendments essentially codified practices of testing and manufacturing that were already being used by the medical device industry.

The introduction of the CON system and of rate regulation in some states did affect the diffusion of some costly medical devices (see the paper by Hillman in this volume). Basically, however, the market continued to be driven by new technology, and the physician in a hospital setting remained the major buying influence. As before, the medical profession had, in effect, few financial constraints on the adoption and use of medical technology. As a result, during these years the rate of growth of the medical devices industry continued to be healthy.

PUBLIC POLICY AND MEDICAL DEVICES: 1983 TO THE PRESENT

Then, in the fall of 1983, everything changed with the introduction of the Prospective Payment System for Medicare inhospital services based on DRGs. PPS set a national payment rate for hospital care by classifying patients into DRGs that have specific, predetermined reimbursement values, based on the relative resource consumption of the care provided. Payment is determined by this weight and a subsequent adjustment for factors such as the nature of the hospital and local wage rates (Institute of Medicine, 1990). Those familiar with a business environment can appreciate the dra-

---

[1] This statistic should be viewed in context because the calculation was based on the residual method. That is, health care expenditures are regressed against a number of variables (e.g., labor, supplies, facilities) that influence supply and demand for health services. The unexplained residual is then attributed to the use of medical technologies.

matic change that occurred. The health care sector changed from a cost-plus system, in which to make a dollar, a dollar had to be spent, to an administered, fixed-price system—what some might consider a 180-degree turn. The years following 1983 saw the rise of managed care, preferred provider organizations, and, finally, the recent introduction of a physician payment system founded on resource-based relative value scales (RBRVS). For the first time, the medical device industry felt the hand of government not only in the arena of safety and efficacy regulation but in the field of payment strategies.

In the years before 1983, the primary market for medical devices was the in-patient hospital setting, in which the majority of diagnostic and therapeutic interventions were carried out. Beginning in 1983, however, in response to the changes in payment methods noted above, there was a striking shift in behavior. To avoid the capitation imposed by DRGs and CONs in the hospital setting, providers moved to outpatient settings and began to explore alternative methods of service delivery (e.g., mobile scanning units). The results were soon apparent. Between 1976 and 1990, outpatient visits to community hospitals increased more than 64 percent, to 326 million visits per year. In the same period, outpatient visits per 1,000 Blue Cross subscribers increased 114 percent. Hospital-based ambulatory surgeries grew about 108 percent between 1983 and 1989. A look at more recent trends reveals that seasonally adjusted outpatient visits to community hospitals increased to 84 million visits in the first quarter of 1991, up 44 percent from the same quarter in 1985 (*Hospitals*, 1991). There are predictions that this trend will continue and that hospital outpatient activities will grow from levels of about 16 percent of all hospital income in 1985 to at least 25 percent of income by the year 2000 (Premier Hospitals Alliance).

By 1987, hospitals had begun to adjust to the new payment realities. Some continued to try to maximize revenue by buying sophisticated equipment that helped recruit physicians, who in turn attracted patients. But it soon became clear to forward-looking hospital administrators that the pursuit of revenue was not the only answer to their budgetary problems and that indulging in nostalgic longing for the bygone days of cost-plus payment was an idle pastime. Lowering costs, increasing productivity, and improving outcomes were seen as ways to improve the hospital's financial position. In particular, hospitals began to manage their costs more closely. Speculation among its developers that PPS would lead to the discontinuation of unprofitable services proved unfounded. Rather, hospitals added services in an attempt to increase profitability by attracting cases that were known to be potentially profitable. Their goals were to increase their market share and to shift their payer mix to any remaining cost-based payers (Prospective Payment Assessment Commission, 1989).

In addition to these shifts in the health care economy, two potentially major policy changes are under discussion. The first is the introduction of so-called user fees, a mechanism by which industry itself would underwrite the funds needed by the FDA to process premarketing approval (PMA) requests[2] and premarketing notifications or 510(k)s.[3] One suggestion is to charge $100,000 for each application sent to the FDA. The second policy change is to tie payment to clinical evidence that a new technology improves patient health or lowers costs. To qualify for payment, manufacturers would have to prove to the satisfaction of a third party that their devices meet these objectives. These changes, in combination with the trends noted above, may have a significant effect on the medical device industry and its R&D strategies.

Such an effect will be felt in an industry that has been under substantial pressure for the past decade. During the period following 1983, the market experienced what economists call a stochastic shock—a change of monumental proportions. When DRGs were implemented the market suffered a major drop in its compound average growth rate, and the single-digit growth rates that were seen following the drop continued to the present. In 1984, the industry experienced negative growth for the first time in its history. Thus, despite some of the adjustments made by providers to continue to acquire promising new medical technologies, PPS had the desired effect of slowing the flow of capital equipment into the health care market.

Implications for Medical Device R&D

The changes that occurred in the policy environment in this period, in conjunction with advances in the knowledge base underlying device development, affected the kinds of technologies that were developed. What resulted was a medical device market of greatly increased complexity that exhibited the classic fragmentation of a mature market. The traditional product category of physician aids remained, but expanding engineering capabilities created new options for diagnosing and screening. Dramatic new imaging modalities, such as cardiovascular ultrasound, allowed cardiologists for the first time to look at moving structures in the heart. Cineangiography appeared in the catheterization labs; computed tomography (CT) scanners and MRI gave physicians the ability to look at physiological structures in ways that had scarcely seemed possible a decade previously.

---

[2] Under the requirement for premarketing approval the device manufacturer must provide reasonable assurance of safety and effectiveness under the conditions of intended use.

[3] To obtain premarketing notification, also known as a 510(k), the manufacturer must present evidence that its device is substantially equivalent to an earlier, approved device. If the device is not substantially equivalent, it cannot be marketed until a PMA is approved or the device is reclassified.

The growing importance of liability concerns in U.S. health care also affected device development. Those involved in liability issues in the medical community, in their efforts to control rising malpractice rates, discovered that information, in the form of well-documented events, constituted a better defense for liability than a string of character references. Products appeared on the market whose main purpose was to provide accurate, valid information in the case of potential liability. Storage and Recall Obstetrical Management Systems were introduced that can retain a fetal monitoring strip for 23 years. Gas monitoring in the operating room, motivated in large part by liability concerns, became common. With such innovations in technology and practice, the liability insurance for anesthesiology has gone down dramatically. Documentation systems in the operating room and in the intensive care unit (ICU) are other examples of recently introduced information technologies.

The current trend is to move beyond the mere documenting of information and to use that information to actually improve the process of care. This movement to measure results and outcomes has stimulated the development of such products as clinical information systems, which make it easier for a physician to compare real outcomes with predicted ones to determine whether a procedure makes a difference. Clinical information systems that collect primary data in the ICU are one example, as are scoring systems such as APACHE and TISS.

As a greater premium is placed on providing cost-effective care and shorter hospital lengths of stay, incentives have increased for manufacturers to develop technologies that enable care to be moved to alternative, lower-cost outpatient settings. Innovative developments such as catheterization labs, angioplasty, and intraocular lens implants are driven to a great degree by the payment system, as is the production of imaging devices that can be moved about in a mobile van.

Another trend—patient preferences—has begun to exert a stronger influence on R&D than in the past as the medical device industry responds to the growing importance of patient involvement in determining the use of particular diagnostic or therapeutic interventions. Previously, the patient was fairly isolated from choice. Now, in designing devices, particularly for healthy persons, the industry gives greater consideration to the user—for example, in the case of Holter monitors, to whether the device is comfortable to wear. In the case of MRI and CT technologies, there are other patient comfort, as well as access, issues to consider: whether the banging "noise" is bothersome or whether the closeness of equipment produces claustrophobia. The new Lucile Salter Packard Children's Hospital at Stanford has wired one-and-a-half floors for Hewlett-Packard telemetry—a communications lifeline that permits toddlers, for example, unsupervised freedom of movement (instead of being confined to their cribs) at the same time vital life signs are being monitored. Noninvasive sensors such as pulse oximetry and automatic blood pressure cuffs improve both comfort and safety (Gerard, 1991). Such products are a tangible demonstration of the industry's increased level of concern about patient preferences and comfort in the design of new devices.

In addition, device manufacturers are starting to invest more heavily in studies that show that their products improve outcomes or decrease costs. For example, according to a recent study on the effectiveness of Hewlett-Packard bedside computers in intensive-care nursing, ICU nurses can now spend 22 percent less time recording data; this time savings frees them to perform more nursing care at the bedside and improves a hospital's efficiency. In fact, the Lutheran Hospital in La Cross, Wisconsin, where this study took place, has eliminated 6 hours a day of nursing overtime and reduced the nursing staff by one full-time-equivalent position (Allen and Davis, 1991).

In sum, the medical device industry has moved from a rather simple marketplace driven by new technologies and new modalities, to one of multiple patient settings, multiple product categories, and multiple motivations to purchase. The product introduction process has been affected by the addition of the government-introduced regulatory "screens" discussed earlier. Some of these screens have had positive effects on device R&D strategies, but some of the policy changes that are under debate may have less beneficial results. "We are dealing with a market that is defined increasingly by regulation and payment policies rather than by technology, patient needs, and competitive forces" notes Jerry E. Robertson, executive vice president and general manager, Life Sciences Sector, 3M Corporation (Robertson, 1990).

To appreciate the potentially negative impact of the introduction of user fees (see the previous discussion), several unique characteristics of the industry must be understood. There are 16,000 medical device companies registered with the FDA. These are mainly small companies, among which sales are not evenly distributed. For example, the top 50, or one-third, of these firms account for 95 percent of sales. In the particular case of prosthesis manufacturers, 7 percent of the companies account for 50 percent of sales. Frequently, small firms are the early-stage innovators who bring new modalities to the market (Roberts, 1988), which are then produced and distributed on a broader scale by larger manufacturers. This process occurs because it is characteristic of the medical device market that once a new modality is introduced, it can be copied with relative ease. Innovation thus occurs in increments within the various firms, with the first introduction of a product often being the result of development by the small companies.

To return to the issue of user fees, the law stipulates that a PMA must be completed within 180 days; in reality, the average review cycle is about

415 days. The burden of user fees if enacted, in both time and money, would be particularly onerous to small firms. The average development time of a product in a lab is 18 months to 2 years. To be required to invest $100,000 and also experience a significant time delay at the end of that process would jeopardize the ability of these small companies to innovate and commercialize rapidly.

The success of the U.S. device industry depends on small firms bringing innovation quickly to the market and legislators must protect this capability. Obviously, a larger company is better able to manage such fees and to survive delays in time to market, but history has shown them to be less likely to produce new technologies. In conclusion, user fees related to PMAs and 510(k)s and the delays that may result in seeking approval for marketing are potentially harmful and could impede the ability of the medical device industry to bring innovation to the marketplace.

In addition, the increasingly stringent requirements of insurers and providers for evidence that a new device improves outcomes or lowers costs may have some drawbacks. It is extremely difficult to fully assess a medical device before its introduction into use. Often, as an innovation is used in clinical practice over a period of time, it reveals possibilities that were not envisioned by its originators. Many product successes were completely unforeseen at the time of market introduction. The following examples demonstrate that the clinical world is, in fact, a laboratory as technology diffuses.

S. James Adelstein, now executive dean for academic programs of the Faculty of Medicine at Harvard Medical School, was a practicing radiologist at the time of the introduction of the CT scanner. He asked his associates to fill out two slips of paper, which were sealed in an envelope that would be opened 5 years later. He asked them to answer two questions: What is a CT scanner good for today? and Will it be used in 5 years? "What was most striking," Adelstein said after opening the envelopes 5 years later, "was not the errors of commission but those of omission" (S. J. Adelstein, Harvard Medical School, personal communication December 12, 1991).

Good examples of the continuing innovation that occurs following a product's initial diffusion are also available from Hewlett-Packard (HP). The company entered the ultrasound field in the early 1960s with a product that looked for deviations in the midline of the brain induced by trauma—but there was only a limited market for the product. In 1981 the firm introduced a cardiovascular system based on that initial device, which has been quite successful—a situation that was not easy to predict given HP's first entry into the market and the way that the technology initially was used. HP was also one of the first firms to introduce an oximeter in 1978. It was an ear oximeter for use in sleep studies (a small market) and sold for about $12,000. Seven or eight years later, with the development of pulse oximetry, the market grew to what is now a $150 million business. Today, pulse oximeters are a major factor in preventing hypoxia (an oxygen deprivation of the brain caused by improper anesthesia). The March 31, 1991, edition of the *Boston Globe* summarizes the current environment:

> Using techniques developed at the Harvard hospitals and a new piece of equipment called a pulse oximeter, a small device worn on the finger that emits a signal when the flow of oxygen drops, doctors have all but relegated hypoxia to the dustbin of medical history. Thus, life has improved for patients and anesthesiologists, whose annual malpractice premiums have fallen to under $9,000 a year from $25,000 in just four years.

When HP first introduced its ear oximetry technology, no one could have predicted this use, nor the dramatic contribution it would make. The incremental innovation demonstrated in the above examples is important, however, and payment schemes should not unnecessarily restrict the evolution of medical devices within clinical practice.

OBSERVATIONS

Recognizing the interplay of these various regulatory and payment interventions, how should the medical device industry respond? One way to view the problem is from the perspective of the fourth quadrant of the Cartesian coordinate system (see Figure 13-1). This is where I believe the medical device industry needs to focus its product development efforts to design products that do one of two things: either improve outcomes or help keep the cost of health care down—or, ideally, yield the vector sum of both these endpoints. Everything the industry does must pass muster as lying along one of those two axes.

In addition, the industry must work to rid the health care arena of frivolous, redundant technological modalities that drive up costs but provide no counterbalancing benefits. It must discourage overutilization of its products. For the electromedical industry to continue to innovate, it must also educate policymakers regarding the fundamental distinction between the invention of technology and its utilization. All too often, the virtues of invention are being blamed for the sins of overuse and inappropriate use.

Without question, the industry can be attentive to lowering overall health care costs. Yet it should be kept in mind that the development of new medical devices is a particularly costly and risky enterprise. As a group, U.S. medical technology companies invest as much as 6.2 percent of their sales revenues in R&D—but many spend as much as 15 percent or more. These figures become even more pointed when compared with the national average for U.S. manufacturers, which is 3 percent of sales. When a medi-

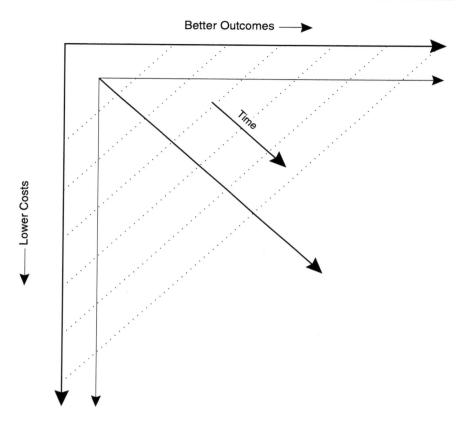

FIGURE 13-1 Fourth quadrant in a Cartesian graph of costs and outcomes.

cal device firm introduces a product, it needs to know what it must do to satisfy government regulations and how long it will take to get approvals. In an uncertain regulatory environment, companies face increased risks with innovation (Health Industry Manufacturers Association, 1991).

Today, a company could wait months or years to find out whether a new technology will be approved for marketing and whether the costs for its use will be reimbursed. (It took several years, for example, before MRI received approvals.) It is unrealistic to expect firms, especially small ones, to support a product through what could be quite lengthy approval cycles. We must continue to explore a middle ground, in which some technologies would be covered earlier or on an interim basis while they are undergoing further evaluation. This approach could address both access and utilization concerns while retaining incentives for innovation.

In conclusion, the device industry has seen dramatic change over the past 27 years, and further policy change seems likely. Despite some financial buffeting, the electromedical device industry remains a profitable enterprise, which produces a $3.2 billion positive balance of trade and employs about 248,000 Americans (Bowles, 1990). Its continued strength and ability to support innovation is likely to lead to improvements in existing products and the capability to address emerging health care needs.

What is done in the coming years to reshape the health care system in this country will affect the products that the industry is able to develop and produce, and will help to define the kind of medical interventions that will be available in the decades ahead. I am confident that industry, government, and health care providers can, in the spirit of collaboration, generate solutions that will create a more cost-effective health care system that will not unnecessarily hamper innovation.

REFERENCES

Allen, D., and Davis, M. 1991. *Clinical Information Systems Impact on the Intensive Care Unit.* La Crosse, Wisc.: Lutheran Hospital. March.

Altman, S. H., and Rodwin, M. A. 1988. Halfway competitive markets and ineffective regulation: The American health care system. *Journal of Health Politics, Policy and Law*, 13(2):323-339.

Bowles, J. 1990. America's miracle industry. *Fortune*, December 17.

Gerard, B. 1991. Medical marvels. *Measure*, September-October, pp. 16-19.

Health Industry Manufacturers Association. 1991. *Competitiveness of the U.S. Health Care Technology Industry.* Washington, D.C.: The Association, pp. H19-H20.

Hospitals. 1991. Tracking the long-term growth in outpatient care. Vol. 65, issue no. 23, p. 16.

Institute of Medicine. 1990. *Medicare: A Strategy for Quality Assurance.* Vol. 1. K. N. Lohr, ed. Washington, D.C.: National Academy Press, pp. 108-109.

Office of Technology Assessment, U.S. Congress. 1984. *Medical Technology and Costs of the Medicare Program.* Publication No. OTA-H-228. Washington, D.C.: Government Printing Office.

Premier Hospitals Alliance. *Setting the Alliance Standard Premier's Strategic Plan—1991.* Chicago, Ill.: Premier Hospitals Alliance, p. 15.

Prospective Payment Assessment Commission. 1989. *Medicare Prospective Payment and the American Health Care System—Report to the Congress.* Washington, D.C.: Prospective Payment Assessment Commission, June, pp. 112-113.

Roberts, E. B. 1988. Technological innovation and medical devices. In: *New Medical Devices: Invention, Development, and Use.* Washington, D.C.: National Academy Press, p. 46.

Robertson, J. 1990. The future of HIMA: Taking the longer view. Presentation at the Annual Meeting of Health Industry Manufacturers Association. March 20.

Shabot, M. M. 1990. *Changing Policies for Reimbursement of Surgeons: Impact on the Introduction and Use of Technologies in the Surgical ICU.* Los Angeles, Calif.: Cedars-Sinai Medical Center, p. 4.

14

The Changing Health Care Economy: Impact on Surgical Techniques

Frank G. Moody

The complexity of surgical therapy and its demand for life-saving and life-supporting technology have made it especially vulnerable to reductions in the nation's investment in biomedical research and development. In fact, improvement in the safety and efficacy of surgical therapy depends critically on continued evolution of more sophisticated technology and techniques for the diagnosis and treatment of those diseases amenable to operative manipulation. Cost factors, however, that in part relate to successes derived from the application of innovative technologies have generated a critical assessment of therapies that require an extraordinary use of health resources (Showstack et al., 1985). Organ transplantation, coronary artery bypass, hip replacement, and multimodal cancer therapy are only a few examples of treatments commonly used in the United States but applied with restraint elsewhere in the world because of their expense.

Of equal importance is the question of the public good. Because money has emerged as a rate-limiting step in the application of new technologies abroad, it is reasonable to assume that the continued inflation of the health dollar in the United States will lead to similar concerns and restraints in the future application of expensive therapies. The rapid movement of surgical treatment from the hospital to the outpatient setting is an indication that surgeons are responding to the forces of the marketplace. But what effect will this traditionally free-enterprise adaptive response have on future innovation? Will surgeons abandon their quest for cures of some of humanity's most devastating diseases? I do not believe so, but in a way, surgeons have become the victims of their own success in applying the remarkable technological advances that characterize the latter half of this century.

The following treatise relates the day-to-day practice of surgery to the current health care scene. It examines surgical mores and provides an explanation as to why surgical therapies have remained relatively unfettered by bureaucratic regulation. It also discusses surgery's use and possibly misuse of technology. Finally, it offers an example of a feedback loop in real time in which technology leads to new techniques that in turn lead to new technology, and so forth. The process repeats itself for the betterment of the patient—but at a price. This paper attempts to establish a construct that will convince the reader that investments in innovative technology in the present will produce not only social benefits but cost savings in the future.

THE SURGEON AS INNOVATOR

Surgery is a therapeutic discipline that has its origins in the inherent physical violence of ancient times. Not much has changed over the centuries; war and its need for aggressive treatment of the wounded have stimulated many modern advances in surgical therapy. The need for timely interventions to control bleeding, remove fragments of missiles, and excise nonviable tissue or body parts provided the beginnings for a bold, often daring, yet risky medical discipline that, for the most part, depends on ingenious manipulative approaches to the problems it attempts to resolve.

One of the earliest and most effective therapies for a common civilian ailment was the "cutting of the stone" (in medical terms, the removal of a bladder stone by perineal cystotomy) (Barrey, 1933). One can hardly imagine the pain of the stone and the pain of the incision in the era before anesthetics and analgesia. It is no wonder that surgeons were by necessity itinerant and poorly regarded by their medical colleagues. Furthermore, operative procedures such as perineal cystotomy were associated with postoperative morbidity that sometimes was worse than the disease.

From the beginning, surgeons were innovative, because patients presented for treatment with their own particular manifestations of disease and anatomical deformities. What might be a satisfactory operative approach for one patient could be disastrous for another with the same disease.

This author finds it helpful to distinguish novel therapies from innovative therapies. A novel procedure is one that has never been done before; innovative therapies are those that are successful over time and are adopted into general practice. The independent nature of surgical practice in this country has allowed the development and application of a variety of successful techniques. Operations on the heart, the brain, the liver, and other vital organs stand as marvels of modern medicine (Ravitch, 1981). In academic and urban medical centers, transplantation of organs, excision of cataracts, joint replacements, and endoscopic and interventional radiologic techniques are part of everyday practice. These advances came about because of the need to help someone with a life-threatening or life-limiting ailment. Some of the other critical factors in surgical innovation are ideas, technology, evaluation, regulation, liability, and money. Translating the ideas that are generated, in response to patient needs, into effective, safe therapies depends on a process of technological development, which includes evaluation as an essential component.

The remarkable advances made in surgical therapy during the past several decades are in part a result of the relatively unregulated environment of surgical practice. Indeed, during the early days of the development of modern surgical techniques, the only regulation came from the limits of technology. Surgical treatment was a personal contract for service between the surgeon and the patient; the service required only an operating room, an anesthesiologist, the operating team, and some relatively simple tools. Often, the use of innovative therapies were attempts to correct or improve desperate, often life-threatening problems for patients for whom the trip to the operating room was the path of last resort. Liability was not a major consideration, nor was money, because payers reimbursed charges for the new and ultimately life-saving therapies. A climate of fiscal constraint, however, has made money, liability, evaluation, and regulation the dominant considerations at the end of this remarkable period of medical history. The emphasis now being placed on these factors may constrain the development of new therapies. Nevertheless, there remains a need for new ideas and for continuing evolution of all aspects of medical technology.

THE CURRENT STATUS OF SURGICAL INNOVATION

There is little evidence up to this point that the pace of innovation in surgery has changed during a decade characterized by obsession with the rising costs of health care. Nevertheless, as commentators elsewhere have noted, other aspects of health care have been significantly affected. This section discusses some of the implications for surgical innovation of current trends in the health care industry.

The two major payers in the health delivery system, industry and government, are tightly bound in a synergistic relationship. The components of our society that provide the wherewithal to care for patients' needs might best be called a health care industry. Pharmaceutical houses, device makers, software packagers, clinics, hospitals, publishers, third-party payers, physicians and other health workers, and educational institutions are all important elements of the health care industry. Major changes in the activities of one component will have a profound effect on the functions of the others. The defense industry provides a good analogy in its diverse relationships with various segments of the economy.

As noted earlier, innovation in surgical practice is intimately linked to advances in drugs and devices. Examples abound: synthetic prostheses and sutures, the heart-lung machine, antibiotics, parenteral nutrition, and immunosuppressive agents, to name only a few. To be useful, innovation must have an application. Surgeons on occasion perform novel procedures, but unless the procedure, through application and refinement, can be shown to be effective and safe, it will not be accepted into practice in the long run. Unfortunately, many procedures are put into practice prior to rigorous evaluation of clinical and economic outcomes. Recognition of this shortcoming has led to an increasing emphasis on outcome research, as has been discussed elsewhere (Wennberg, 1990).

The process of cost analysis is quite foreign to surgeons who, as a group, are accustomed to the high costs of their procedures and who tend to employ whatever tools or techniques might help their patients, regardless of their cost. One of the reasons for such an attitude is that surgeons are often called upon to render therapy in the advanced stages of a disease. Organ transplants, for example, are not usually performed until the patient's organ fails. Severely injured patients often require extensive interventions and prolonged stays in the intensive care unit if they are to survive, and even treatments of this type may fail after expenditures of hundreds of thousands of dollars. Until recently, the true costs of therapy have been difficult to assess, but diagnosis-related groups (DRGs) introduced a strong incentive to do so. Hospitals have quickly learned how to distinguish charges from costs, because their very survival depends on careful financial analysis. Surgeons and physicians in general have been slow to appreciate the costs they impose on the system, but recent discussions of changes in reimbursement through the resource-based relative value scale (RBRVS) have stimulated a high level of awareness with regard to the relative worth of professional service. The cost-effectiveness of surgical therapy raises the question of endpoints. Is a therapy effective when it provides a few months or years of useful life, but the patient dies of the disease for which he or she is treated? Is cosmetic surgery cost-effective? Should older patients be denied the benefits of coronary bypass surgery because their days are already numbered? These are issues that must be addressed by the public and the profession in the years ahead.

Surgeons appear to be adaptable and have quickly learned to comply with Medicare's prospective payment system and its method of reimbursing hospitals by DRGs (Schwartz and Mendelsen, 1991). Following implementation of the DRGs, lengths of stay for surgical patients dropped precipitously, and surgical procedures rapidly moved from the hospital to the ambulatory setting. Patients were no longer admitted for preoperative workups, and even patients facing complex surgical procedures went directly from home to the operating room after only a brief stay in a preoperative staging area. This shift from inpatient to outpatient performance of procedures, however, did not appear to alter the rate of escalation of the aggregate cost of surgical care, although, in fact, it appears that surgical care was improved. The financial success of an ambulatory surgicenter requires careful cost accounting and a well-managed business environment. Efforts thus were made to accomplish surgical procedures in a more cost-effective, efficient manner.

ASSESSMENT OF NEW PROCEDURES

Surgeons have been slow to incorporate rigorous assessment of their procedures into their culture (Wennberg et al., 1988). Other areas of medicine, however, have used randomized controlled trials to determine which of two or more alternative therapies might be the best approach to a specific disease. The current trials of carotid endarterectomy versus medical therapy are a good example of an instance in which subpopulations of patients who might benefit from a surgical approach were identified (North American Symptomatic Carotid Endarterectomy Trial Collaborators, 1991). Controlled trials have also shown the efficacy of approaches to treating breast cancer that are less morbid than surgery but equally effective (Berté et al., 1988). Controlled trials to determine whether surgical therapy is better than medical therapy are uncommon. Nevertheless, advances in pharmacological approaches to what previously were thought to be exclusively surgical problems (e.g., prostatism, complications of peptic ulcer disease, hyperthyroidism) have rapidly displaced commonly performed surgical procedures. Clearly, effective, less invasive therapies are preferred over surgical procedures by patients and practitioners, even though surgery may be more definitive in resolving the problem. When type 2 histamine (H-2) blocking agents became available to control the symptoms of peptic ulcer, there was no need for a randomized trial to establish the superiority of the medical versus the operative approach. Until the introduction of potent antisecretory agents, a surgical approach was the only way to relieve the intolerable and sometimes life-threatening manifestations of a duodenal or gastric ulcer. The less morbid and equally effective pharmacological therapy has emerged as the treatment of choice for the uncomplicated form of this common disease.

In general, the outcomes of randomized trials usually reveal a lack of superiority of one surgical therapy combined with another or with a nonsurgical option. There are many reasons for this—for example, the diversity of the disease being treated and its varying manifestations in different subjects. It is also difficult to control the conditions of the trial and ensure that only the variable of interest is being measured; the need to conduct the trial at multiple sites and to use different surgeons in order to recruit an adequate number of patients over a reasonable period of time can introduce a great deal of variability.

Portasystemic shunting for the prevention of esophageal hemorrhage from portal hypertension is an example of the complexity involved in applying controlled trials to surgical treatment (Resnick et al., 1974). The idea certainly had merit: preventing variceal hemorrhage would greatly reduce the morbidity of this serious complication of portal hypertension. But what was learned in the trial was that, although a portasystemic shunt significantly reduced the risk of esophageal hemorrhage, it increased the rate of death from liver failure. Furthermore, some patients who probably would never have bled from their varices died of liver failure as a consequence of the procedure (Rikkers, 1982). Subsequent advances in therapy, however, sometimes render former studies of little contemporary relevance, and this proved to be the case here (Rikkers, 1990). Variceal scleral therapy has recently emerged as a less invasive, more effective way to control bleeding of esophageal varices in most patients, and liver transplantation has replaced portasystemic shunting for patients with a failing liver, even among alcoholic patients. Social concerns, however, have constrained the application of this expensive, organ-limited procedure among alcoholic patients (Cello et al., 1987; Kumar et al., 1990).

ARE THE COSTS AND BENEFITS OF NEW SURGICAL PROCEDURES CALCULABLE?

The incremental cost of introducing a new surgical procedure is gradually assuming critical importance. For example, if third-party payers will compensate hospitals or physicians only for well-established therapies, it is unlikely that new treatments, even if less costly or more effective, will be utilized. Current Procedural Terminology (CPT) codes establish what procedures payers, private as well as public, will cover. The shift from the "usual and customary" compensation base to a "relative value" fee schedule may also serve to determine which operations are done. In addition, if payers only cover operations that have proven efficacy and safety in the hands of the doer, a tightly controlled system will evolve that may be better for the individual patient but that will significantly constrain a surgeon from exercising his or her judgment. A system of this kind would require a large body of normative experience and detailed validation of outcome criteria as a reference. Furthermore, it assumes that the patient populations being treated are homogeneous, which is far from the truth in most complex diseases. One potential outcome of such a system might be that therapeutic decisions based on and limited to fee schedules would have a dampening effect on surgical innovation, because the decision would fail to recognize procedures that have not been proved effective.

The new order of health care cost management must find a way to allow well-trained surgeons to provide services to those who need them with a minimum of bureaucratic interference. It appears that the introduction of the prospective payment system, of utilization review and second opinions, and even of managed care has not significantly influenced the types of operations that are performed or the kinds of patients who undergo them. What surgeons do for their patients is governed by the usual process of graduate surgical education, postgraduate courses, journals, and professional meetings. Schemes that are designed to limit the application of surgical options at the point of service are not likely to be effective. They can only slow down the application of treatment at the time it is needed, not prevent its use if it is the best or only option.

The denial of surgical service because of lack of access based on financial considerations is another concern. Refusing payment for the performance of a gastric restrictive procedure for chronic morbid obesity is a case in point. In spite of the availability of two safe, reasonably effective operations for this debilitating disease—the vertical-banded gastroplasty and the small-pouch Roux limb gastric bypass—public and private insurers have markedly restricted the benefits of these operations by refusing to cover them. The recent consensus conference sponsored by the National Institutes of Health attested to the unique benefits of these procedures and may correct this injustice to those with a genetic predisposition for morbid obesity (National Institutes of Health, 1991).

Decisions about which treatments should be offered to patients must be made by those professionals who understand the patient and his or her illness and life situation. Such important, highly individualized decisions cannot easily or even appropriately be made by a committee, either locally or in Washington. The issues of appropriateness of care and level of control of therapeutic decision making are complicated by the nation's third-party reimbursement system. If the patient was more directly involved in purchasing surgical services, the patient-surgeon procedural contract could be a bilateral negotiation, but such is not the case. Payers have an increasing interest in controlling the treatment options offered to their patients. This is a positive trend if the exclusive point of service is selected on the basis of established proficiency rather than on costs alone.

THE COST-EFFECTIVENESS OF INNOVATION

Unfortunately, the individualized doctor-patient relationship has not prevented, and may be a factor in, the increases that have occurred in the cost of medical care over the past two decades. Physicians have always been the purveyors of health services for their patients, and only recently have they become sensitive to the limitations of the system they broker. The incremental rise in health expenditures parallels the opportunities for precision in diagnosis and treatment. Innovative technology has brought medicine to the point of being able to treat afflictions that previously were thought to be uncorrectable. It is unfortunate that the lack of money, whether in the form of federal or state budgets, the profit margins of industry, personal financial resources, or a percentage of the gross national product, should be the major rate-limiting step to further improvements in health care. The U.S. health care system is simply too expensive and not uniformly accessible to all who live in this country. Total expenditures for health care in 1992 are estimated to be in excess of $700 billion; if used wisely, these funds should be enough to deliver a high level of health care to all U.S. residents.

Although money is not the only important variable in a health care system, it is at the center of current discussions. Thus, the question of costs and their relationship to innovative therapies must be considered. Will new procedures that are effective and applicable to large numbers of patients increase or reduce the cost of treating a specific disease? It is difficult to assess the aggregate cost of a therapy for the country at large because of marked regional differences in charges for hospitalization and services.

Let us compare the costs of a minimally invasive procedure—transluminal angioplasty—and an operative approach—coronary bypass—to those of a common serious disease, myocardial infarction (Wittels et al., 1990). An angioplasty and its follow-up over 5 years cost approximately $27,000, compared with $32,500 for coronary bypass surgery. The absolute numbers are not important except to acknowledge that such studies can be done; what these studies do not reveal, however, is the cost to society if the disease had been left untreated. Each procedure has shown efficacy in selected patients; thus it is likely that such studies will be done with the modern tools of cost analysis. The cost savings as a result of an earlier death are likely to favor nontreatment—a frightening thought as health care researchers attempt to develop cost-effectiveness algorithms. Perhaps a better way to assess the benefits of costly therapies is to compare the cost of a therapy that is definitive in curing a disease with another that supports the management of a chronic disease. Such studies of the treatment of end-stage renal disease have been done and have even reached the halls of Congress. Congressman Fortney "Pete" Stark of California's 9th District and chair of the House of Representatives Subcommittee on Health recently stated that "each successful (renal) transplant saved Medicare $19,656 per year per patient."[1] Again, the numbers are not important; what is important is that data derived from clinico-economic studies have reached key decision makers in Congress.

Cost-benefit analysis should be targeted toward the benefits that will be gained from continued improvement in definitive therapy and the potential benefits to be derived from the knowledge acquired through research and development. The treatment of end-stage diseases will always be expensive (Garner and Dardis, 1987); thus, it was thought that prevention of costly disease processes would be the only hope for decreasing the rate of increase in health expenditures in the years ahead. Recent studies, however, have suggested that prevention may not necessarily lead to cost-reducing effects (Russell, 1986).

THE CASE OF GALLSTONES

To address more specifically the issue of cost containment and surgical intervention, this section considers the dramatic changes that are occurring in the treatment of gallstones, a common, easily quantifiable disease (Roslyn and DenBesten, 1990). It is estimated that more than 20 million people in the United States have gallstones. In addition, a million new cases are identified each year. Several unique features of gallstones should be borne in mind. First, if the stones stay within the lumen of the gallbladder, the patient usually does not know that they are there. Indeed, approximately half of the people with gallstones are asymptomatic; only 15 percent will suffer a potentially life-threatening complication. The most common complaint is that of severe right-sided upper abdominal pain, a symptom called biliary colic. Once a patient with gallstones has biliary colic, he or she is likely to have subsequent episodes, which denote the passage of stones from the gallbladder. Such patients are then at risk of developing the severe complications of acute cholecystitis, cholangitis, and gallstone pancreatitis.

Until a few years ago, the only definitive treatment of symptomatic gallstones was removal of the gallbladder through an incision in the abdomen, a procedure called a cholecystectomy (McSherry, 1989). An improved understanding of the pathogenesis of cholesterol gallstones, the most common stones seen in Western countries, has led to several alternatives to this type of surgery: (1) oral dissolution, (2) direct dissolution, (3) lithotripsy, and (4) lithotomy. Simultaneously with improved understanding of the

---

[1] In a letter dated September 13, 1991, Congressman Stark writes: "I'm not sure where I made the comment on the savings to Medicare of successful transplants, but it sounds right for the pre-EPO [erythropoietin] period. The figure is obviously higher now, by about $4,000, and will be rising further as the composite rate is gradually adjusted for inflation." Quoted with permission.

origins of gallstones have come dramatic advances in the ability to image and access the gallbladder and the biliary tree. Ultrasound, computer-assisted scanning, percutaneous transhepatic cholangiography, and endoscopic retrograde cholangiography have offered new approaches to the treatment of gallstones and their sequelae.

Treatment options for symptomatic gallstones now range from simply taking two pills a day to removal of the gallbladder. Because therapies that leave the gallbladder in place have a recurrence rate of 20 to 50 percent, it could be argued that the gallbladder should be removed in all patients who are symptomatic. But operative removal of the gallbladder is not without its risks of death (0.2–1.0 percent) and of postoperative complications and pain. Moreover, the cost of hospitalization (5–7 days) is about $5,000 and is followed by a relatively long period of recovery (2–3 weeks). As one might expect, physicians and patients found the alternatives to surgery attractive when they were introduced several years ago; on the other hand, general surgeons were not particularly pleased, given that the alternative treatments represented a potential loss of income by decreasing the volume of one of the most common procedures they performed.

This description should provide sufficient background to understand what has happened to these newer, less invasive therapies and how their use involves interplay with the medical profession, the research establishment (the National Institutes of Health and industry), regulatory bodies (the Food and Drug Administration and other public agencies), and third-party payers, public and private. Oral dissolution, the least invasive of the various therapies, is also the most limited in its therapeutic efficacy (Fromm, 1986). Ursodeoxycholic acid (ursodiol), the bile salt used for this purpose, is almost without side effects but it only dissolves small stones, preferably those that are single, noncalcified, and floating, characteristics that suggest a high concentration of cholesterol. Larger, noncalcified stones can be fragmented by extracorporeal shock wave lithotripsy, a procedure that focuses the energy of sound waves generated outside the body on a gallstone or stones (Sackmann et al., 1988). Residual fragments that the body does not pass spontaneously are dissolved with ursodiol.

Oral dissolution, with or without lithotripsy, is time-consuming and requires the ingestion of ursodiol for several months or, in some cases, years. This type of therapy is ineffective in noncompliant patients and unpopular in a health delivery system that is concerned with costs and immediate results. Lithotripsy for gallstones, although initially promising, has not fulfilled the expectations of patients, physicians, and the regulating bodies concerned with efficacy and cost of the technology. Some lithotripters cost more than $1.5 million to purchase and install. Trials of this innovative therapy have been initiated but are currently incomplete. It appears that at one year retention of residual fragments even with bile salt therapy is such that this form of therapy must be considered relatively cost-ineffective. Nevertheless, there may be a subpopulation of patients with gallstones that could be cured either by lithotripsy alone or by a combination of lithotripsy and oral dissolution.

Direct dissolution of gallstones by the instillation of methyl tert-butyl ether, a liquid at body temperature, is also a relatively effective treatment (Thistle et al., 1989). Among its advantages are that it requires no general anesthesia and only a brief stay in the hospital; it also has the potential to treat a larger stone burden than can be treated by oral dissolution with or without lithotripsy. The technique, however, is time-consuming, tedious, invasive (although minimally so), and potentially toxic.

THE SYNERGISM OF NEW TECHNOLOGY

The enthusiasm for developing alternatives to cholecystectomy has been dramatically tempered by a recent surgical innovation, laparoscopic cholecystectomy, which involves the removal of the gallbladder through small puncture wounds made at appropriate sites in the upper abdomen. The technique requires tubular entry ports for a camera and the operative instruments; the procedure is then performed by visualizing the operative manipulations on a television screen. This approach has rapidly replaced open cholecystectomy for the treatment of symptomatic gallstones, and its development has greatly reduced interest in alternatives to cholecystectomy (Reddick and Olsen, 1989).

An analysis of the interplay between these competing innovative therapies reveals several unique characteristics of the current health care scene. For example, surgeons adopted and perfected the laparoscopic approach to cholecystectomy so rapidly that the device industry found itself incapable of satisfying demand for the devices. The public learned of the potential of the procedure through the media before most surgeons were aware that a cholecystectomy could be done in this less invasive way. Yet within months, surgeons were learning the technique and utilizing it in their practices. Its popularity derives from its shorter hospital stay (only overnight) and a much shorter period of recovery compared with open cholecystectomy; in addition, the small incisions required in the procedure are much less painful and disfiguring. Thousands of laparoscopic cholecystectomies have been performed since the first use of the procedure in 1987. Its rapid displacement of open cholecystectomy is somewhat surprising, because it requires general anesthesia, takes longer to perform, has a higher rate of bile duct injury, and results in comparable mortality (Peters et al., 1991). Possibly its high rate of adoption in everyday surgical practice derives from the relative lack of success of the alternatives when tested in formal clinical trials. Another factor may be the frustration of general surgeons who were forced to sit on the sidelines during the evaluation, often by nonsurgeons, of these potentially less invasive ways to treat gallstones as patients were entered into clinical trials.

THE DYNAMICS OF INNOVATION

The recent evolution of treatments for gallstone disease emphasizes the interplay of public demand, payers' preferences for less costly alternatives to cholecystectomy, professional interest, and innovation. Lithotripsy for the treatment of gallstones has fallen out of favor because of its great expense and the problem of fragment retention. Oral dissolution by the ingestion of ursodiol, although safe, is effective in only a small number of patients who have small (<3 mm) floating gallstones. Percutaneous dissolution has not progressed beyond early phases of development. All of the alternatives to cholecystectomy have been superseded by the current enthusiasm for laparoscopic cholecystectomy, a procedure that has been adopted into surgical practice without formal evaluation and assessment of outcome. With this new technique, surgical treatment is again the treatment of choice for the majority of patients with symptomatic gallstones. There remains a small group of patients who might benefit from alternative treatments—for example, patients who are at risk of associated medical problems if anesthetized. The elderly, who have the highest incidence of gallstones as well as the greatest risk from their complications, might also benefit from a minimally invasive, yet effective, approach to their problem. It is in this population that oral and direct dissolution with or without lithotripsy may play a role. These techniques, however, are limited in their application because, as noted earlier, they are effective only in patients with cholesterol gallstones and are best suited to patients with small stone burdens.

Advances in the field are continuing; a recent example currently under evaluation is a device called a lithotrite. The lithotrite can be placed into the gallbladder lumen through a small puncture wound in the skin using local anesthesia (Miller et al., 1991). Interventional radiologists who are experienced in percutaneous transhepatic cholangiography, a commonly performed procedure, can use the lithotrite with a high level of precision and safety. The lithotrite consists of a metal basket, small at its base, with a propeller, or impeller, as it is called. Rotations of the impeller at a rate of between 20,000 and 30,000 revolutions per minute create a vortex that draws gallstones into the basket and leads to their rapid pulverization. The debris is then drained from the gallbladder, and after irrigation, its lumen is examined by contrast radiography to demonstrate stone clearance. The device is unique in that it can fragment cholesterol as well as noncholesterol and calcified stones and thereby clear the gallbladder of stones with a single treatment and without general anesthesia. In preliminary trials, it appears to be not only safe but effective in the hands of biliary interventional radiologists.

Advances in technology have a remarkable interactive synergy. For example, the lithotrite has been adapted for use by surgeons to gain stone clearance from the gallbladder during performance of a laparoscopic cholecystectomy. The ultimate worth of this technology will not be known until controlled trials are conducted. Even at this early stage of assessment, however, researchers have learned that the device will not accommodate large stones. The fragmentation of large stones by lithotripsy may offer a way to further extend the applicability of the lithotrite. The device may also solve the main problem associated with direct dissolution and lithotripsy: clearance of residual fragments from the gallbladder. The lithotrite emphasizes how novel techniques may enhance the usefulness of older therapies that during their own evaluations were found to be lacking in effectiveness. It also highlights the complexities involved in predicting the usefulness of novel technology.

SUMMATION

The current focus on the costs of health care is likely to continue into the next century as the United States attempts to deal with the complex illnesses of an ever-larger aging population. Life expectancy in the not too distant future will approach 100 years, and it is projected that there will be one elderly adult (>65) for each child by the turn of the century. It is imperative that we continue to seek new approaches to old problems and to adapt technology to the task. Although prevention of disease is the goal being sought, the realities and consequences of disease as it exists in each patient must nevertheless be addressed. There should be little argument with the concept that the treatment for each patient should be the one that is most effective and safest. Thus, risk-benefit ratios should take precedence over cost-effectiveness concerns; cost-effectiveness analysis should include an assessment not only of the immediate outcome and the financial resources required to accomplish it but of the ultimate impact of the resolution of the problem as it relates to future general costs and benefits to society.

Managed care, for better or for worse, is growing in popularity as a solution to the rising cost of health care. At issue is whether controls will be applied at the site of care or at some central point by the establishment of general budgets for service centers, such as exists in Canada. The way surgery is practiced in this country would be significantly—and probably negatively—affected by the latter kind of system, because the volume of services would be restricted by the dollars available in the budget. The American public has become accustomed to receiving the benefits of modern health care in a timely fashion. Unfortunately, the sheer expense of providing the ultimate in therapy on demand has denied a large segment of our population access to even the basic rudiments of medical care.

Specialization has provided surgeons a way to perfect their skills and to develop techniques for treating complex problems. If carried to an extreme, however, it could deprive the public of broadly trained physicians who have the breadth of knowledge and skills to treat the majority of conditions that occur in most communities.

With regard to innovation and the development of innovative therapies, specialization and its demands for new products are the driving forces behind the development of safer, more effective, and more cost-effective therapies. As outcomes research is further refined and applied to the assessment of surgical results, it is likely that specialized services will be regionalized. Cardiac surgery, trauma care, and organ transplantation have already moved in that direction, and it is likely in the future that the treatment of severe abnormalities of other organ systems will follow suit.

Optimism is needed during this transition from an inefficient, highly personalized, and relatively expensive health care delivery system to one that with further refinements in surgical techniques and knowledge of the origins of disease will lead to a healthier, more productive population. The increased availability of public and private funds that would result from better health of the citizenry should go far in covering the expense of maintaining the health of those living in this country; the development of more effective, safer surgical techniques would clearly contribute to achieving this goal. Economic considerations and their political implications should not be allowed to be a major deterrent to the health of a nation as richly endowed with human and physical resources as the United States.

REFERENCES

Barrey, J. D. 1933. Lithiasis. In: B. Lewis, ed. *History of Urology*, vol 2. Baltimore: Williams and Wilkins, pp. 1-25.

Berté, E., Buzdar, A. U., Smith, T. L., and Hortobagyi, G. N. 1988. Bilateral primary breast cancer in patients treated with adjuvant therapy. *American Journal of Clinical Oncology* 11:114-118.

Cello, J. P., Grendell, J. H., Crass, R. A., Weber, T. E., and Trunkey, D. D. 1987. Endoscopic sclerotherapy versus portacaval shunt in patients with severe cirrhosis and acute variceal hemorrhage. *New England Journal of Medicine* 316:11-15.

Fromm, H. 1986. Gallstone dissolution therapy. Current states and future prospects. *Gastroenterology*. 91:1560-1567.

Garner, T. I., and Dardis, R. 1987. Cost-effectiveness analysis of end-stage renal disease treatments. *Medical Care* 25:25-34.

Kumar, S., Stauber, R. E., Gavaler, J. S., Basista, M. H., Dindzans, V. J., Schade, R. R., et al. 1990. Orthotopic liver transplantation for alcoholic liver disease. *Hepatology* 11:159-164.

McSherry, C. K. 1989. Cholecystectomy: The gold standard. *American Journal of Surgery* 158:174-178.

Miller, F. J., Rose, S. C., Buchi, K. N., Hunter, J. G., Nash, J. E., and Kensey, K. R. 1991. Percutaneous rotational contact biliary lithotripsy: Initial clinical results with the Kensey Nash lithotrite. *Radiology* 178:781-785.

National Institutes of Health. 1991. *Consensus Statement for Gastrointestinal Surgery for Severe Obesity.* Bethesda, Md.: Office of Medical Applications of Research.

North American Symptomatic Carotid Endarterectomy Trial Collaborators. 1991. Beneficial effect of carotid endarterectomy in symptomatic patients with high-grade carotid stenosis. *New England Journal of Medicine* 325:445-453.

Peters, J. H., Ellison, E. C., Innes, J. T., Liss, J. L., Nichols, K. E., Lomano, J. M., et al. 1991. Safety and efficacy of laparoscopic cholecystectomy. *Annals of Surgery* 213:3-12.

Ravitch, M. M. 1981. *A Century of Surgery: The History of the American Surgical Association.* Philadelphia: J. Lippincott.

Reddick, E. J., and Olsen, D. O. 1989. Laparoscopic laser cholecystectomy. *Surgical Endoscopy* 3:131-133.

Resnick, R. H., Iber, F. L., Ishihara, A. M., Chalmers, T. C., and Zimmerman, H. 1974. A controlled study of the therapeutic portacaval shunt. *Gastroenterology* 67:843-857.

Rikkers, L. F. 1982. Operations for management of esophageal variceal hemorrhage. *Western Journal of Medicine* 136:107-121.

Rikkers, L. F. 1990. Portal hypertension. In: F. G. Moody, ed. *Surgical Treatment of Digestive Disease,* 2nd ed. Chicago: Year Book Medical Publishers, pp. 363-380.

Roslyn, J. J., and DenBesten, L. 1990. Gallstones and cholecystitis. In: F. G. Moody, ed. *Surgical Treatment of Digestive Disease,* 2nd ed. Chicago: Year Book Medical Publishers, pp. 253-275.

Russell, L. B. 1986. *Is Prevention Better than Cure?* Washington, D.C.: The Brookings Institution.

Sackmann, M., Delius, M., Sauerbruch, T., Hall, J., Weber, W., Ippisch, E., et al. 1988. Shock-wave lithotripsy of gallstones. *New England Journal of Medicine* 318:393-397.

Schwartz, W. B., and Mendelsen, D. N. 1991. Cost containment in the 1980's. *New England Journal of Medicine* 324:1037-1042.

Showstack, J. A., Stone, M. H., and Schroeder, S. A. 1985. The role of changing clinical practices in the rising costs of hospital care. *New England Journal of Medicine* 313:1201-1207.

Thistle, J. L., May, G. R., Bender, C. E., Williams, W. J., Leroy, A. J., Nelson, P. E., et al. 1989. Dissolution of cholesterol gallbladder stones by methyl tert-butyl ether administered by percutaneous transhepatic catheter. *New England Journal of Medicine* 320:633-639.

Wennberg, J. E. 1990. What is outcomes research? In: A. C. Gelijns, ed. *Medical Innovation at the Crossroads.* Vol. 1, *Modern Methods of Clinical Investigation.* Washington, D.C.: National Academy Press, pp. 33-46.

Wennberg, J. E., Mulley, A. G., Jr., Hanley, D., Timothy, R. P., Fowler, F. J., Jr., Roos, N. P., et al. 1988. An assessment of prostatectomy for benign urinary tract obstruction. *Journal of the American Medical Association* 259:3027-3030.

Wittels, E. H., Hay, J. W., and Gotto, A. M., Jr. 1990. Medical costs of coronary artery disease in the United States. *American Journal of Cardiology* 65:432-440.

Part VII
Concluding Observations

15

Summing Up:
Reflections on Medical Innovation and
Health Care Reform

Harvey V. Fineberg

Americans seem to have an ongoing love-hate relationship with medical technology. We manage somehow to hold two contradictory views—seeing technology as the culprit behind rising medical care costs and as the jewel in the crown of American medicine. This dual characterization—technology as both hero and villain—underlies this collection of papers exploring the direction of health care reform and its likely impact on the process of medical innovation. The authors in this volume appear to disagree more over the desired locus of managerial control in such reform than over its likely effect on medical innovation. Fundamentally, all are motivated by a laudable, though elusive, objective: to preserve investment in and progress toward needed medical advances while stifling technology that is harmful or that costs more than it is worth.

As escalating medical costs threaten the security of growing numbers of middle-class Americans, reform in the financing of U.S. health care takes on heightened political expectations. Two critical elements of reform are broader, more secure insurance coverage for all Americans and reliable mechanisms for containing the growth in health care costs. The great debate, of course, is over the all-important details and unintended consequences: Who shall bear the costs, and how shall they be distributed? What mix of public and private financing mechanisms will work best and be most acceptable? What means of cost control will be least onerous and still get the job done? What is the proper balance between market forces and regulation as mechanisms for resource allocation? How can the quality of care be maintained and sensitivity to patient needs strengthened? And, the question directly prompting this volume, how will the process of medical innovation fare in the new age of health care reform?

As explained in Chapter 1, medical technology covers a wide spectrum of drugs, devices, equipment, practices, and support structures. The model of medical innovation summarized by Laubach, Wennberg, and Gelijns suggests that the process of innovation occurs in diverse settings and ways. The practicing physician and surgeon shape the use of drugs, devices, and instruments as surely as the research chemist in a pharmaceutical firm or the engineer in an equipment manufacturing company. If we are to comprehend the effects of health care reform on medical innovation, then we must comprehend not only the varieties of potential reform, but the impact of these reforms on a multiplicity of actors, including patients, practitioners, institutional providers, entrepreneurs, drug companies, and device and equipment manufacturers.

The precise nature of financial and programmatic reform in the U.S. health care system is under active debate. The authors in this volume differ on the level at which "management" control should ideally be exercised in the new health care system. Some (such as Soper and Ferriss) hail the advantages of what has come to be known in the United States as managed care, believing that it offers the potential for higher quality of care, improved patient satisfaction, and better allocation of resources. Others (such as Wennberg) proclaim the virtues of system-level controls and lament the dangers—especially those arising from ignorance of what truly works in medical care—of attempting to regulate decisions at the level of individual practitioners. Wagner advances a model of management that stresses an intermediate, institutional level, seeing the health maintenance organization as a means of integrating a population perspective and operational capacity for control of resource use.

From the vantage point of the patient, Mulley argues that a deeper danger in rigid clinical decision rules is their neglect of personal values that may make all the difference in choosing courses of diagnosis and treatment. This type of criticism may also be applied to the formulaic approach being pursued in the Oregon ranking system described by Welch and Fisher.

In the course of their discussion of the Canadian health care system, Barer and Evans point out that all health systems ration and manage care. To an economist, rationing occurs whenever a resource is finite, and the term does not connote the image of deprivation that it conveys in everyday use. In its current health care system, the United States does make choices, often by default, about resource allocation and management control. The debate about reform in U.S. health care makes a number of these choices more evident and explicit. What, for example, will be the degree of reliance on market forces and competition among health care providers and payers? What will be the nature and mechanisms of management control at systemwide, institutional, and individual practitioner levels? How will the interests of individual patients and communities be incorporated in medical care decisions?

In contemplating health care reform, it is easy—and wrong—to confuse what creates a problem with what exposes the problem. The Oregon ranking system described by Welch and Fisher did not create rationing of medical services among the state's Medicaid population. Efforts to make medical decision making more systematic did not create ignorance about health outcomes and other consequences of medical interventions. Attempts to incorporate patient values and preferences into treatment decisions did not create insensitive clinicians. The issue in each case is to identify root causes of the problem and to devise ways to ameliorate them.

From the other countries' experience with their health systems, we may derive three pertinent lessons. First, universal coverage may be attained in a single-payer system (such as Great Britain's) or in a multipayer system (such as Germany's). Second, universal coverage alone does not ensure cost control. Third, even the combination of universal coverage and cost control does not guarantee that resource allocation decisions will be made rationally or after careful evaluation. Williams, for example, points out in his paper that the United Kingdom has failed thus far to guide the diffusion of medical technology in a purposeful way.

We in the United States have come to expect advances in medical technology almost as a matter of course: miracle drugs, better laboratory tests, new ways of harnessing energy to visualize anatomic structures, creative use of space-age materials, innovative techniques in surgery, and electronic monitoring marvels. Such advances do not occur as a matter of routine, but result from a confluence of science, investment, talent, motivation, and opportunity.

The richness of the crosscutting discussion in this volume about health system reforms and their implications should not obscure a fundamental, underlying truth: *Any system of payment for health care exerts a profound influence on the pace and direction of medical innovation.*

Current incentives for investment in medical care are far from ideal. If we spend a great deal of money on insurance systems and documentation, we can expect entrepreneurs to invest effort and money in developing more creative and effective tools to extract payments based on whatever rules of reimbursement are in place. If hospitals compete by marketing their services to overlapping communities of patients, then, as Griner notes of the experience in Rochester, we may expect those hospitals to acquire equipment or offer services that will provide a perceived competitive advantage (while meeting patient needs). Hillman draws similar conclusions in his description of physician decisions to acquire and use new technology. Such investments make perfectly good sense from the vantage point of a hospital or other provider, even if neither promises any real advantage to patients or communities.

Whatever the complete mix of ingredients that determine medical innovation—from cultural values to scientific advances to serendipity—there can be little doubt that innovation in the form of new medical products is subject to the same economic forces that apply in any commercial field of endeavor. Capital investment tends to flow over time to fields offering the greatest expected return on investment, and expectations of economic return will ultimately determine the amount of capital drawn to the health field. Although medical technology typically is shaped and reshaped by practitioners, capital investment in new ventures and established companies remains the principal engine behind new product innovation.

The costs of medical care to a payer also represent income to a provider and return on investment to a supplier. On the face of it, the process of new product innovation seems imperiled by reforms that would diminish growth in payments for medical services. Two factors, however, diminish this hazard. First, even with lower rates of growth, the medical care sector is sufficiently large as to present significant opportunities for economic return on investment. Second, as discussed in the chapters by Telling and Holmes, pharmaceutical makers and equipment manufacturers are able and willing to respond to new economic incentives through such strategies as emphasizing development of more cost-effective alternatives and by reaching for truly breakthrough products. In this connection, Laubach, Wennberg, and Gelijns note the several innovations in less costly or ambulatory practice (such as lithotripsy) that have emerged from European companies and practitioners, where the rates of growth in medical costs have been temperate compared to those in the United States. Quite possibly, the new emphasis on cost-effective and breakthrough innovations (along with slowing of the rise in their own medical insurance costs) will position U.S. manufacturers to compete even more effectively in the global medical market.

Thinking optimistically, what may emerge from health care reform is an enlightened strategy for medical innovation that responds to population health needs, to new system and organizational requirements, and to significant advances in biological and technical knowledge. From the various recommendations posed throughout this volume, I would in closing highlight three: an ethic of evaluation, education of physicians and patients, and public policy to promote innovation.

By an ethic of evaluation, I mean a widespread commitment and expectation among physicians, health care institutions, and the public that medical practices must be evaluated for effectiveness, safety, and cost. At the heart of this new ethic is a recognition of how little is known about the consequences of many medical interventions, whether new or well established in practice. Adopting a systematic, pervasive strategy for evaluation will require public and private resources, but the return in terms of extended lives, reduced suffering, and cost savings can be substantial.

Many leading medical educators are pursuing educational reforms that would better prepare physicians to understand the family and community context of their patients, the importance of disease prevention, the changing nature of the medical care system, scientific advances pertinent to clinical practice, and their roles as problem solvers in partnership with patients and as lifetime learners. Among the many challenges to medical education is to nurture an experimental outlook and desire for improvement of the sort that, for example, animated the stream of surgical advances described by Dr. Moody. If we expect physicians to be sensitive to the phenomenon of their patients' illnesses, as expressed so eloquently by Mr. Silberman, they must be taught how to do so. Physicians who can combine a heightened level of sensitivity to patients, technical skill, willingness to experiment, and commitment to evaluation will be valuable players in the new era of health care reform.

Finally, innovation in medical care can be stimulated by expanded public investment in basic biomedical research, tax and other economic incentives that favor investment in companies developing new technology, and fresh approaches in such regulatory bodies as the Food and Drug Administration to facilitate experimentation and earlier, controlled dissemination of technology (perhaps coupled with more stringent postmarketing evaluation requirements). Ideally, these policies would serve to accelerate the pace of innovation while steering the health care system toward cost-effective and genuinely advantageous technology.

While the precise nature of reforms in health care remains to be seen, this volume launches a constructive dialogue on the probable consequences for the process of medical innovation. The discussion is likely to continue for some time and should be better informed because of this effort.

Appendixes

A

Workshop Agenda

Improving the Translation of Research Findings into Clinical Practice: Workshop III

THE CHANGING HEALTH CARE ECONOMY: IMPACT ON PHYSICIANS, PATIENTS, AND INNOVATORS

April 18, 1991

8:00 a.m. *Registration and Continental Breakfast*

8:30 a.m. **Welcome and Opening Remarks**
William Hubbard, Committee on
Technological Innovation in Medicine

8:45 a.m. **Keynote Address: The Changing Health Care Economy**
John Wennberg, Chair of Workshop III,
Dartmouth College

9:15   a.m.   **A Reaction**—Uwe Reinhardt, Princeton University

9:30   a.m.   Discussion

9:45   a.m.   *Break*

Session I: **Changes in the Financing and Delivery of**
                     Health Services
                     Moderator: Susan Bartlett Foote,
                        Robert Wood Johnson Fellow

10:15   a.m.   **The Growth of Managed Care in the Private Sector**
              Michael Soper, CIGNA
              David Ferriss (co-author), CIGNA

10:45   a.m.   **A Reaction—The Experience with HMOs**
              Edward Wagner, Group Health Cooperative of Puget Sound

11:00   a.m.   **Managing Care and Capacity in the Public Sector:**
              The United Kingdom
              Alan Williams, York University, United Kingdom

11:30   a.m.   **The Meeting of the Twain: Managing Health Care**
              Capital, Capacity, and Costs in Canada
              Morris Barer, University of British Columbia, Canada
              Robert Evans (co-author), University of British Columbia,
                 Canada

12:00   a.m.   **A Reaction—Public-Sector Mechanisms in Medicaid:**
              Oregon's Priority List
              Gilbert Welch, Dartmouth College

12:15   p.m.   Discussion

1:15   p.m.   *Lunch*

Session II: **Changes in the Diffusion of New Technology:**
                     The Provider's Perspective
                     Moderator: Jerome Grossman, New England Medical Center

2:00	p.m.	**The Hospital and Changes in the Adoption of New Technology** Paul Griner, Strong Memorial Hospital
2:30	p.m.	**Physicians' Acquisition and Use of Technology** Bruce Hillman, University of Arizona
3:00	p.m.	*Break*
3:15	p.m.	**Provider Panel Discussion:** Alan Nelson, Memorial Medical Center, Salt Lake City, Utah Paul Barrett, Kaiser Permanente, Denver, Colorado Mary Mundinger, Columbia University Arnold Aberman, University of Toronto
5:00	p.m.	Discussion
5:30	p.m.	*Adjournment and Reception*

April 19, 1991

8:00	a.m.	*Continental Breakfast*
8:30	a.m.	Opening by John Wennberg, Chair of Workshop III, Dartmouth College
Session III:		**Changes in the Diffusion of Technology:** **The Patient's Perspective** *Moderator*: John Wennberg, Dartmouth College
8:45	a.m.	**The Patient's Stake in the Changing Health Care Economy** Albert Mulley, Massachusetts General Hospital
9:15	a.m.	**What Is It Like to be a Patient in the 1990s?** Charles Silberman, New York City
9:45	a.m.	Discussion
10:30	a.m.	*Break*

Session IV: **Changes in the Development of New Medical Technology**
                   Moderator: Gerald Laubach, Chair, Committee on Technological Innovation in Medicine

10:45   a.m.   **Industrial Strategies for Pharmaceutical Research and Development**
                   Frederick Telling, Pfizer Pharmaceuticals
                   Barry Bloom (co-author), Pfizer Pharmaceuticals

11:15   a.m.   **Industrial Strategies for Medical Device Development**
                   Ben Holmes, Hewlett-Packard

11:45   a.m.   Discussion

12:15   p.m.   *Lunch*

1:00   p.m.   **Surgical Techniques Originating in Academic Health Centers**
                   Frank Moody, University of Texas Health Science Center, Houston

1:30   p.m.   Discussion

2:30   p.m.   **Summing Up: Medical Technology and the Changing Economics of Health Care**
                   Harvey Fineberg, Harvard University

3:00   p.m.   *Adjournment*

B

Contributors

MORRIS L. BARER is director of the Centre for Health Services and Policy Research and a professor in the Department of Health Care and Epidemiology at the University of British Columbia. He is also an associate of the Centre for Health Economics and Policy Analysis at McMaster University and an associate of the Canadian Institute for Advanced Research, Program in Population Health. He presently serves as the senior editor for health economics of *Social Science and Medicine*. Dr. Barer has conducted research and published widely in the areas of physician resource policy; trends in health care utilization, particularly among the elderly in British Columbia; comparative health care system funding and organization; and comparisons of health care costs and use in Canada and the United States. Recent papers have appeared in *The Milbank Quarterly, New England Journal of Medicine, Journal of Health Politics, Policy and Law, International Journal of Health Services, Health Services Research, Inquiry,* and the *Canadian Medical Association Journal.* He is also a co-author of two recent research monographs—*The Growth in Use of Health Services, 1977/78 to 1985/86,* published by Saskatchewan Health, and *Australian Private Medicare Care Costs and Use, 1976 and 1986,* published by the Australian Institute of Health—and a major policy report, *Toward Integrated Medical Resource Policies for Canada,* published by the Canadian Conference of Deputy Ministers of Health.

ROBERT G. EVANS is an internationally known expert on the economics of health care, an active participant in developing policies for the Canadian health care system, and a health care consultant in Europe, Asia, and the United States. A graduate of the University of Toronto in political economy, he earned a Ph.D. in economics from Harvard University in 1970; he is currently professor of economics at the University of British Columbia, Vancouver, where he has been a faculty member since 1969. He was a member of the British Columbia Royal Commission on Health Care and Cost, which has recently issued its final report, and is currently a member of the main advisory committee for the National Health Research and Development Program. He is also a faculty member of the Centre for Health Services and Policy Research at the University of British Columbia and an associate member of the Centre for Health Economics and Policy Analysis at McMaster University. He was president of the Canadian Health Economics Research Association from 1983 to 1986 and is a fellow of the Canadian Institute for Advanced Research and director of the Institute's Program in Population Health.

DAVID M. FERRISS, JR. is associate national medical director for the CIGNA Employee Benefits Division. Dr. Ferriss earned his M.D. from Tulane Medical School in 1976 and his M.P.H. in health services from the University of California, Los Angeles, in 1981. He is a diplomate of the American Board of Family Practice and the American Board of Preventive Medicine. Dr. Ferriss joined CIGNA in 1985 and served for three years as the medical director of CIGNA Healthplan of Colorado. He assumed his present position in CIGNA's National Medical Department in 1990, following a two-year leave of absence during which he was a postdoctoral fellow in health services research at the Johns Hopkins University School of Hygiene and Public Health.

HARVEY V. FINEBERG received his A.B. degree from Harvard University in 1967, his M.D. from Harvard Medical School in 1972, and his Ph.D. from the John F. Kennedy School of Government in 1980. Dr. Fineberg is dean of the Harvard School of Public Health; prior to his appointment to that post in 1984, he was a professor in health policy and management at the Harvard School of Public Health. Dean Fineberg has been a leading figure in the health policy field. As a member of the Public Health Council of Massachusetts from 1976 to 1979, he participated in decision making on matters of hospital investment and health policy. From 1982 to 1985, he served as chairman of the Health Care Technology Study Section of the National Center for Health Services Research. Dean Fineberg's past research has focused on several areas of health policy, including the process of policy development and implementation, assessment of medical technology, and dissemination of medical innovations. He helped found and has served as president of the Society for Medical Decision Making.

Dr. Fineberg is a co-author of two books: *Clinical Decision Analysis* and an analysis of the controversial federal immunization program against the swine flu in 1976, *The Epidemic That Never Was.* He is the author of numerous journal articles, including the recent "Education to Prevent AIDS: Prospects and Obstacles" in *Science* and "The Social Dimensions of AIDS" in *Scientific American.* He is a member of the Institute of Medicine (IOM) and served on the IOM committee that produced the report *Confronting AIDS* in 1986. In 1988 he received the Joseph W. Mountin Prize from the epidemiology section of the American Public Health Association. He is also a member of the board of directors of the American Foundation for AIDS Research and has served as a consultant to the World Health Organization.

ELLIOTT S. FISHER is an assistant professor in the Departments of Medicine and of Community and Family Medicine at Dartmouth Medical School and is part of the medical staff of the White River Junction Veterans Administration (VA) Hospital. He is a graduate of Harvard College and the Harvard Medical School. Dr. Fisher completed his residency training in internal medicine at the University of Washington where he was also a fellow in the Robert Wood Johnson Clinical Scholars Program. His principle research interests are in health policy and the use of large data bases for research. His research includes comparisons of surgical outcomes in the United States and Canada and comparisons of VA and private health care system effectiveness.

ANNETINE C. GELIJNS joined the Institute of Medicine (IOM) as an international fellow and is now director of the Program on Technological Innovation in Medicine. Before joining the IOM, she was senior researcher for the Project on Future Health Care Technology, cosponsored by the European office of the World Health Organization (WHO) and the Dutch government. From 1983 to 1985, Dr. Gelijns worked for the Steering Committee on Future Health Scenarios, where she helped develop models for long-term health planning in the areas of cancer, cardiovascular disease, and aging; she also had a joint appointment to the Staff Bureau for Health Policy Development, Department of Health, the Netherlands. She has been a consultant to various national and international organizations, including the WHO and the Organization for Economic Cooperation and Development. She is a member of the board of the International Society on Technology Assessment in Health Care. Her research interests focus on medical innovation, and she has authored a number of publications on the subject, including a recent book on the dynamics of medical technology development. She received the LL.M. degree from the University of Leyden and her Ph.D. from the University of Amsterdam.

PAUL F. GRINER, who holds the academic title of Samuel E. Durand Professor of Medicine at the University of Rochester School of Medicine, has been general director of Strong Memorial Hospital since March 1984. A graduate of Harvard College, Dr. Griner received his M.D. degree, with honors, from the University of Rochester School of Medicine and Dentistry. He completed an internship and residency in medicine at the Massachusetts General Hospital and served as medical chief resident at Strong Memorial Hospital. In 1964, he was appointed instructor in medicine and a fellow in hematology, and has been a member of the Rochester medical faculty since that time. As the chief executive officer of Strong Memorial Hospital, Dr. Griner is responsible for directing its activities and programs, including its ambulatory services. He also directs the hospital's relationships with the community and with local, state, and federal regulatory bodies. As a nationally recognized authority on medical decision making and the delivery of health care, Dr. Griner has published and lectured extensively on improving the efficiency and effectiveness of clinical practice, the relationship between managerial and clinical decision making in the hospital, and future directions in medicine. He is active in many professional organizations, including the American College of Physicians, where he chairs the Board of Regents. Dr. Griner is a member of the Institute of Medicine, the Association of American Medical Colleges, and the Academic Medical Center Consortium. He has also been appointed to the New York State Governor's Health Care Advisory Board and chairs its Quality of Care and Regulatory Review Committee.

BRUCE J. HILLMAN attended Princeton University, receiving a B.A. degree in 1969, and the University of Rochester School of Medicine, from which he received the M.D. degree in 1973. After finishing radiology training in 1978, which included a one-year research fellowship at the Shields Warren Research Laboratories of Harvard University and specialization in genitourinary radiology, Dr. Hillman became assistant professor of radiology at the University of Arizona; he was promoted to associate professor in 1981 and full professor in 1985, and served as vice chairman of the Department of Radiology from 1986 to 1991. Since 1992, Dr. Hillman has been professor and chairman of the Department of Radiology at the University of Virginia School of Medicine and senior scholar at the University of Virginia Center for Health Policy Research.

During his early career in radiology, Dr. Hillman was awarded George Marshall and John A. Hartford fellowships to pursue his research in renal microcirculation, applications of new technology, and radiologic decision making. In 1984-1985, he was appointed a Pew Foundation Health Policy Career Development Fellow at the RAND/University of California, Los Angeles, Center for Health Policy. Since that time, Dr. Hillman has pursued research dealing with the assessment and diffusion of new imaging technology, competition in medicine, the development of research careers, and new methods for developing practice standards. He is a research consultant to the RAND Corporation, the United Mine Workers Health and Retirement Funds, and the American College of Radiology. Dr. Hillman is editor-in-chief of the journal *Investigative Radiology.*

BEN L. HOLMES is a vice president of Hewlett-Packard Company, a position to which he was appointed in September 1985, and general manager of Hewlett-Packard's Medical Product Group, a position he has held since February 1983. He holds a B.S. degree in applied physics from the University of California, Los Angeles (1959); he received his M.B.A. in marketing from the University of Southern California (1966). A 30-year Hewlett-Packard veteran, Mr. Holmes has held various management positions with the Medical, Computer Systems, and Instruments groups. Previously, he was general manager of Hewlett-Packard's Waltham Division. Currently, he has management responsibility for the design, manufacturing, and marketing of monitoring instrumentation and systems for adults and neonates, diagnostic instrumentation and systems, ambulatory monitoring systems, fetal monitors, ultrasound imaging equipment, health care information systems, and supplies. Mr. Holmes is chairman of the Health Industry Manufacturers Association (HIMA) and a member of the executive committee and board of directors of HIMA and the Massachusetts High Technology Council. He currently serves on the Board of Visitors for Boston University Medical School and is on the IOM Committee on Technological Innovation in Medicine and the Committee on Clinical Evaluation.

GERALD D. LAUBACH holds a B.A. from the University of Pennsylvania and a Ph.D. in organic chemistry from the Massachusetts Institute of Technology. He is formerly president of Pfizer, Inc., and chair of the IOM Committee on Technological Innovation in Medicine. Dr. Laubach is a research chemist by training and served as a laboratory scientist in his early years at Pfizer. He is a member of the Institute of Medicine and the National Academy of Engineering, and served on the now disbanded IOM Council on Health Care Technology. His current activities also include membership on the executive committee of the Council on Competitiveness (successor group to the President's Commission on Industrial Competitiveness), the board of the Food and Drug Law Institute, the Corporation of the Rockefeller University Council, the Carnegie Institution of Washington, the National Committee for Quality Health Care, the Medical Center Advisory Board, the New York Hospital-Cornell Medical Center, and the Corporation Committee for Sponsored Research at the Massachusetts Institute of Technology; he is a director of CIGNA Corporation of Philadelphia and the Millpore Corporation of Bedford, Massachusetts. Previously, Dr. Laubach served as chair of the Pharmaceutical Manufacturers Association from 1977 to 1978 and as a board member until April 1989. He has received honorary doctorates in humane letters from the City University of New York, in law from Connecticut College, and in science from Hofstra University.

FRANK G. MOODY received his M.D. degree in 1956 from Cornell University Medical College. Following a residency in general surgery (1956-1963) at Cornell's New York Hospital, he pursued a research fellowship in gastrointestinal physiology at the University of California Medical Center's Cardiovascular Research Institute in San Francisco. He began his academic career at the University of California Medical Center, followed by appointment to the faculty at the University of Alabama, Birmingham. In 1971, he assumed the chair of surgery at the University of Utah, and subsequently attained his current position as chairman of the Department of Surgery at the University of Texas Medical School at Houston in 1982. Dr. Moody has undertaken more than two dozen visiting lectureships, has been on the editorial board of numerous major journals, is an author of more than 100 peer-reviewed articles, has authored or co-authored 60 chapters in major texts, and has been editor-in-chief or co-editor of 13 books. He has also been president of the American Pancreatic Association, International Biliary Association, Society for Surgery of the Alimentary Tract, and Society of Surgical Chairmen; director of the American Board of Surgery; and chairman of the Council of Academic Societies of the Association of American Medical Colleges.

ALBERT G. MULLEY, JR., is a graduate of Dartmouth College. After receiving degrees in medicine and public policy from Harvard, he completed his residency training in internal medicine at Massachusetts General Hospital. He has remained at Harvard, where he is currently associate professor of medicine and associate professor of health policy, and at Massachusetts General Hospital, where he is chief of the General Internal Medicine Unit. He is the author and editor of *Primary Care Medicine* and of many articles in the medical and health services research literature. Dr. Mulley's research has included the evaluation of intensive care and the cost-effectiveness of prevention strategies and other common clinical practices. Recent work has focused on the use of decision analysis, outcomes research, and preference assessment methods to distinguish between warranted and unwarranted variations in clinical practices. He recently served on the Institute of Medicine Medicare Quality Assurance Committee and is a member of the Clinical Efficacy Subcommittee of the American College of Physicians.

CHARLES E. SILBERMAN is the author of five influential books: *Crisis in Black and White* (1964), *The Myths of Automation* (1966), *Crisis in the Classroom* (1970), *Criminal Violence, Criminal Justice* (1978), and *A Certain People: American Jews and Their Lives Today* (1985). He is currently at work on *Crisis in American Medicine,* to be published by Pantheon Books in 1992. Trained as an economist, Mr. Silberman was a member of the Department of Economics of Columbia University from 1948 to 1953, an associate editor of *Fortune Magazine* from 1953 to 1961, and a member of *Fortune*'s board of editors from 1961 to 1971; he has been a free-lance writer since 1971. Mr. Silberman was awarded the honorary degree Doctor of Human Letters by Kenyon College in May 1972.

MICHAEL R. SOPER is national medical director for CIGNA's Employee Benefits Division, which includes CIGNA Healthplans. He was previously the chief operating officer of AV-MED Health Plan, an independent practice association (IPA)-model health maintenance organization (HMO) in Florida, and the medical director of Prime Health, a staff-model HMO in Kansas City. Dr. Soper has been active with the Group Health Association of America (GHAA) since 1975. He is a past chairman of the Medical Directors' Division of GHAA. Dr. Soper received the M.D. degree, magna cum laude, from Harvard Medical School. His clinical specialty is internal medicine, and he is a fellow of the American College of Physicians.

FREDERICK W. TELLING is vice president, planning and policy, for Pfizer Pharmaceuticals Group. He joined Pfizer in 1977 and held a variety of positions with Pfizer's U.S. pharmaceutical group and its worldwide diagnostic products group, prior to becoming the director of planning for pharmaceuticals in 1981. In 1986, Dr. Telling's responsibilities were expanded to include groupwide public policy issues and medical communications for pharmaceuticals. Dr. Telling graduated from Hamilton College in 1972 with a B.A. in history and economics; he completed a master's degree in industrial and labor relations in 1974 and a Ph.D. in economics and public policy in 1976, both at Cornell University.

EDWARD H. WAGNER is a general internist/epidemiologist and director of the Center for Health Studies at Group Health Cooperative of Puget Sound. He is also professor of health services at the University of Washington School of Public Health and Community Medicine. Previously, he was professor of medicine and epidemiology and deputy director of the Health Services Research Center at the University of North Carolina, Chapel Hill. He is a former member and chairperson of the Health Services Research Study Section of the former National Center for Health Services Research. His current research interests include the evaluation of health promotion/disease prevention interventions, disability prevention in older adults, and the organization of primary care practice.

H. GILBERT WELCH is an assistant professor in the Departments of Medicine and of Community and Family Medicine at Dartmouth Medical School and is on the medical staff at the White River Junction Veterans Administration Hospital. He is a graduate of Harvard College and the University of Cincinnati Medical School. Dr. Welch completed his residency training in internal medicine at the University of Utah and was a fellow in the Robert Wood Johnson Clinical Scholars Program at the University of Washington. He has a strong interest in how resources are best allocated in health care and has authored a number of publications in the area. In particular, he has closely followed the proposed Medicaid expansion in the state of Oregon. Dr. Welch has recently been awarded a Veterans Administration career development grant to study resource allocation methodologies.

JOHN E. WENNBERG is a graduate of Stanford University in California and McGill Medical School in Montreal. He is director of the Center for the Evaluative Clinical Sciences and professor of epidemiology at the Dartmouth Medical School. Dr. Wennberg is a member of the Institute of Medicine (IOM) and serves on a number of national committees including the Health Sciences Policy Board of the IOM and the IOM Committee on Technological Innovation in Medicine. He is the author of numerous publications and is particularly well known for his leading research in small-area variations in health care. He is currently principal investigator for the patient outcomes assessment team (PORT) on prostate disease established under the new federal Agency for Health Care Policy and Research.

ALAN WILLIAMS is professor of economics at the University of York in the United Kingdom. Although for most of his working life he has been an academic economist interested in the appraisal of public expenditures, he also spent two years working inside the Treasury on these same problems, and was a member of the Royal Commission on the National Health Service. He is also a former member of the Department of Health and Social Services Chief Scientist's Research Committee, and the SSRC Health and Health Services Panel. Dr. Williams is a founding member of the United Kingdom Health Economists' Study Group and is director of research projects concerning economic aspects of the care of the elderly, orthopedics, computed tomography scanning, and magnetic resonance imaging. Dr. Williams just completed work on a book with European intensivists that sets out guidelines for the improvement of intensive care in Europe. His current interests are in the measurement of and valuation of health and the economic appraisal of medical technologies; priority setting in the National Health Service, especially the use of cost-benefit criteria; lay concepts of health; the economics of intensive care medicine; the management of waiting lists; technology assessment in health with particular attention to cardiology and radiology; the measurement of patients' quality of life, particularly for patients with epilepsy or multiple sclerosis; the economics of an aging population; and issues of ethical, economic, or clinical freedom.

Index